Your G

GW01388507

Hysterectomy

& *alternative operations*

A GUIDE
TO MENSTRUAL DISORDERS

Jane Smith BSc (Hons)
Medical Editor and Writer, Bristol
&
Alison Bigrigg BM, MRCOG, FRCS, DM
Consultant and Senior Lecturer in Obstetrics and Gynaecology,
University of Bristol, Southmead Hospital, Bristol

ILLUSTRATIONS BY ALEXANDER JAMES

Headway · Hodder & Stoughton

Acknowledgements

We are grateful to many people for their advice and for giving so generously of their time and knowledge, not least to Mr David J. Leaper, FRCS, Consultant and Senior Lecturer in Surgery at Southmead Hospital and the University of Bristol, and to Dr Alasdair Dow, FRCA, Consultant in Anaesthesia and Intensive Care at the Royal Devon and Exeter Hospital.

Thanks are also due to Dr Ian Donaldson, GP; Ward Sister Judy Vickery; Senior Staff Nurse Vanessa McHugh; Superintendent Physiotherapist Sandra Farmer; Mrs Rose West and the staff of The BUPA Hospital Bristol; Mr John Loosley of the Bristol and District Community Health Council; and to Roz, who helped set up the Bristol Hysterectomy Support Network.

We are also grateful to the women who talked to us about their experiences and whose case histories we have used.

British Library Cataloguing in Publication Data

Bigrigg, Alison
Hysterectomy and Alternative Operations.
– (Your Operation Series)
I. Title II. Smith, Jane III. Series
618.1453

ISBN 0 340 62046 3

First published 1994
Impression number   10 9 8 7 6 5 4 3 2 1
Year   1999 1998 1997 1996 1995 1994

Typeset by Wearset, Boldon, Tyne and Wear.
Printed in Great Britain for Hodder & Stoughton Educational, a division of Hodder Headline Plc, 338 Euston Road, London NW1 3BH by Cox & Wyman Ltd, Reading.

Contents

General preface
to the series

Two people having the same operation can have quite different experiences, but one feeling that is common to many is that things might have been easier if they had had a better idea of what to expect. Some people are reluctant to ask questions, and many forget what they are told, sometimes because they are anxious, and sometimes because they do not really understand the explanations they are given.

The emphasis in most medical centres in Britain today is more on patient involvement than at any time in the past. It is now generally accepted that it is important for people to understand what their treatment entails, both in terms of reducing their stress and thus aiding their recovery, and of making their care more straightforward for the medical staff involved.

The books in this series have been written with the aim of giving people comprehensive information about each of the medical conditions covered, about the treatment they are likely to be offered, and about what may happen during their post-operative recovery period. Armed with this knowledge, you should have the confidence to question, and to take part in the decisions made.

Going in to hospital for the first time can be a daunting experience, and therefore the books describe the procedures involved, and identify and explain the roles of the hospital staff with whom you are likely to come into contact.

Anaesthesia is explained in general terms, and the options available for a particular operation are described in each book.

There may be complications following any operation – usually minor but none the less worrying for the person involved – and the common ones are described and explained. Now that less time is spent in hospital following most non-emergency operations, knowing what to expect in the days following surgery, and what to do if a complication does arise, is more important than ever before.

Where relevant, the books include a section of exercises and advice to help you to get back to normal and to deal with the everyday activities which can be difficult or painful in the first few days after an operation.

Doctors and nurses, like members of any profession, use a jargon, and they often forget that many of the terms that are familiar to them are not part of everyday language for most of us. Care has been taken to make the books easily understandable by everyone, and each book has a list of simple explanations of the medical terms you may come across.

Most doctors and nurses are more than willing to explain and to discuss problems with patients, but they often assume that if you do not ask questions, you either do not want to know or you know already. Questions and answers are given in every book to help you to draw up your own list to take with you when you see your GP or consultant.

Each book also has a section of case histories of people who have actually experienced the particular operation themselves. These are included to give you an idea of the problems which can arise, problems which may sometimes seem relatively trivial to others but which can be distressing to those directly concerned.

Although the majority of people are satisfied with the medical care they receive, things can go wrong. If you do feel you need to make a complaint about something that happened, or did not happen, during your treatment, each book has a section which deals in detail with how to go about this.

It was the intention in writing these books to help to take some of the worry out of having an operation. It is not knowing what to expect, and the feeling of being involved in some process over which we have no control, and which we do not fully understand, that makes us anxious. The books in the series *Your Operation* should help to remove some of that anxiety and make you feel less like a car being serviced, and more like part of the team of people who are working together to cure your medical problem and put you back on the road to health.

You may not know *all* there is to know about a particular condition when you have read the book related to it, but you will know more than enough to prepare yourself for your operation. You may decide you do not want to go ahead with surgery. Although this is not the authors' intention, they will be happy that you have been given enough information to feel confident to make your own decision, and to take an active part in your own care. After all, it is *your* operation.

Jane Smith
Bristol, 1994

Other titles published in this series

Breast lumps: A guide to diseases of the breast
Hernias
Varicose veins (published in 1993 by Claremont Press)

Preface

Over 1000 women have a hysterectomy each week in the UK. Many others have an operation to remove the lining of their womb, or start drug treatment in an attempt to control heavy, painful or irregular periods. A hysterectomy is rarely essential for medical reasons: sometimes surgical treatment is necessary for cancer of the uterus or ovaries, but more often it is carried out to improve the quality of life for women who can no longer cope with their menstrual problems, and who may be confined to their homes for a couple of days every month.

There are different types of hysterectomy that can be done, and in some cases women are able to have a say in which one is selected for them. To do so, they must understand what the different operations involve, and what to expect during their recovery period. The book also explains why not all types of operation are suitable for all women.

Although serious complications following a hysterectomy are uncommon, it is a major operation, and it is wise to consider the possible alternatives before opting for this type of treatment.

The aim of this book is to provide all the necessary information and explanations to allow women, where possible, to make their own informed choices.

Jane Smith
Alison Bigrigg
Bristol, 1994

CHAPTER 1

Introduction

A **hysterectomy** is an operation to remove the womb. The operation to remove the ovaries, which may be done at the same time, is called **bilateral salpingo-oophorectomy (BSO)**. A hysterectomy may be carried out to treat menstrual disorders such as heavy, irregular or painful periods. For some women, these symptoms can be dealt with by an operation called **trans-cervical endometrial resection** or **ablation**, in which the endometrial lining of the womb is cut (resected) or burned (ablated) away. For others, drug treatment may be successful, in which case surgery will probably be unnecessary.

Various types of hysterectomy can be performed, depending in part on the reasons for which the operation is being undertaken. To understand what is involved in the various operations, it is necessary to have some knowledge of the structure and normal function of the female genital organs, and these are described in this chapter. Every woman is unique, and different women may have organs of different shapes and sizes.

The internal female genital organs

The internal female genital organs consist of a womb (uterus), two fallopian tubes (uterine tubes), two ovaries, and a vagina. The external opening of the vagina is surrounded by the vulva.

The ovaries

The two ovaries are oval organs which, after puberty, are usually about the size of a walnut (approximately 3 cm long). Each ovary

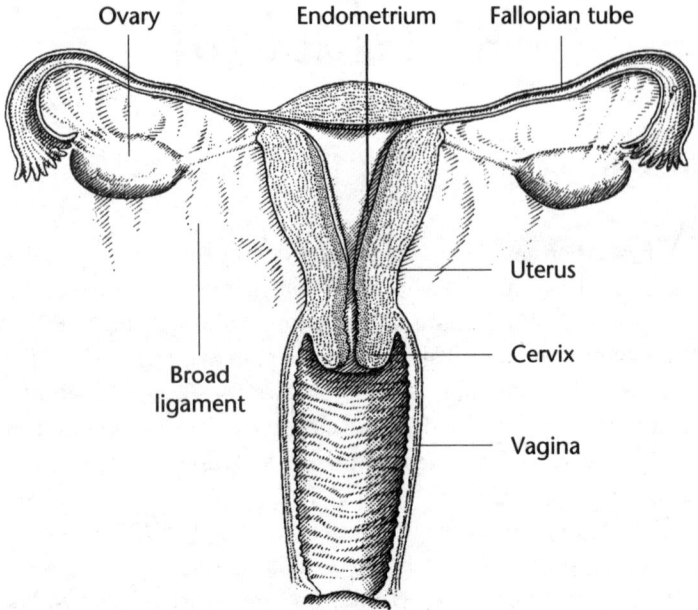

The internal female genital organs.

is situated near the open end of a fallopian tube. The function of the ovaries is to produce hormones and the female eggs, known as **ova** (singular, **ovum**).

Within a newborn baby girl there is a complete complement of several thousand ova, each smaller than a grain of salt. Each ovum is surrounded by a blister-like **follicle**. Although the ova themselves do not increase in size as the girl develops, at puberty some of the follicles mature and enlarge and their ova become surrounded by fluid. At **ovulation**, which normally occurs monthly, in the middle of each menstrual cycle through-out a woman's reproductive life, one of the follicles within an ovary ruptures and releases its ovum. The ovum then passes into the adjacent fallopian tube, and the remains of the follicle form a yellow body known as the **corpus luteum**, which pro-

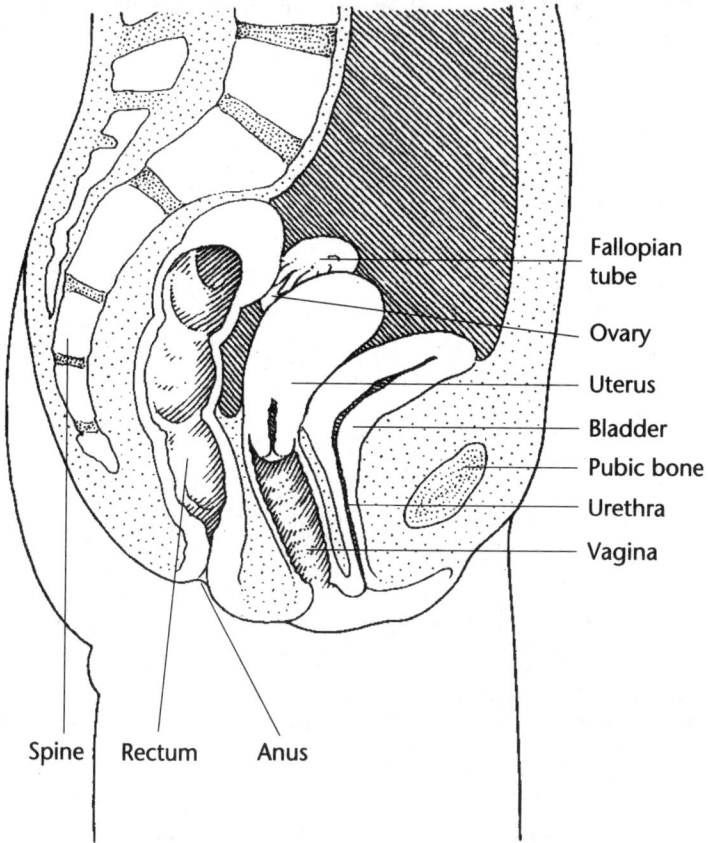

The position of the internal female genital organs in relation to the bladder and rectum.

duces the hormone **progesterone**. Progesterone acts on the lining of the womb to prepare it for pregnancy.

The fallopian tubes

Each of the two fallopian tubes is about the length of a runner bean (on average, approximately 10 cm – 4 inches). The open end of each tube is bordered by tiny hair-like structures which help to waft the ovum into the tube when it is released from the ovary. If an ovum is fertilised by a sperm, the process will normally take place within a fallopian tube, and the fertilised ovum will pass down the tube towards the uterus.

The uterus

The uterus is a muscular organ, about the size and shape of a pear. During pregnancy, it can increase in size by some 30 times. It lies between the bladder and rectum, the bladder being in close contact with its front wall. Because of its proximity to the uterus, the bladder may be affected if the uterus enlarges. For example, if there are fibroids in the uterus (see p. 24), or during pregnancy, the pressure exerted by the enlarged uterus on the bladder may make urination more frequent than normal. The bladder can also be damaged during operations on the uterus itself.

The uterus consists of two main parts: the body, or **corpus**, and the neck, or **cervix**. The fallopian tubes open into its upper corners, the part above which is known as the **fundus**. The cylindrical cervix constitutes the lower part of the uterus where it meets the vagina.

The uterus is rich in blood vessels, and its main function is to provide a suitable, protected environment in which a fetus can develop. During labour, contractions of muscles in the wall of the uterus push the baby down the birth canal.

Secretions from glands within the cervix help to keep the vagina sterile, but during the fertile phase of the menstrual cycle, the alkaline fluid secreted allows penetration by sperm. The cervical canal is normally very narrow, only being wide enough for the passage of sperm and of blood from the uterus during menstruation, but it opens during labour to allow the baby to be born. The cervix itself is very sensitive to stretching.

The uterus has a muscular outer layer, the **myometrium**, and

4

an inner vascular layer, the **endometrium**. The endometrium of a woman during her reproductive life provides a suitable surface for implanatation of a fertilised ovum. During menstruation (see below), bleeding occurs from the many blood vessels of the endometrium, the surface layer of which is then shed. After the menopause (see below), the endometrium and the cervix become thinner and less vascular. As a woman gets older, her uterus shrinks, in most cases to about the size of a chestnut.

The uterus in the majority of women is **anteverted**, i.e. it is angled slightly forwards to curve over the top of the bladder. In some women, however, it is **retroverted**, with its top end angled backwards towards the rectum. Both types are normal, but a doctor who is examining a woman will need to discover, by feeling (see p. 12), which type of uterus she has so that any instrument that is introduced is inserted at the appropriate angle.

The vagina

The vagina is a sensitive muscular canal which extends from the uterus to the vulva. Its length varies from woman to woman, but it is commonly about as long as a pea pod (approximately 8 cm – 3 inches). Its external opening in the vulva is called the **introitus**. The space between the cervix and each wall of the vagina is known as the fornix (plural, **fornices**).

Menarche

The onset of menstruation, known as the **menarche**, normally occurs in girls in the UK between the ages of 10 and 16. This age varies in other parts of the world, being partly dependent on the girl attaining a minimum body weight, and therefore on her level of nutrition.

The menstrual cycle may be irregular to begin with, but usually settles into a pattern after a couple of years.

Menstruation

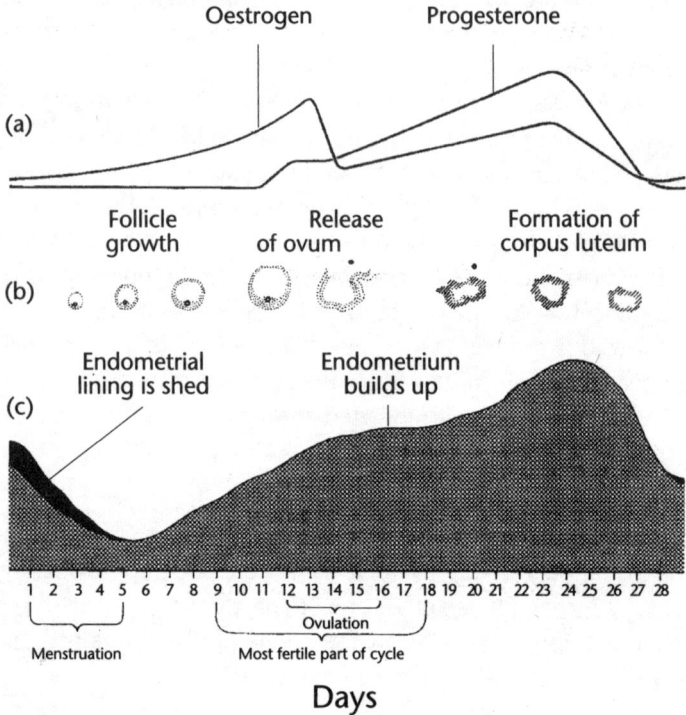

The menstrual cycle. This diagram shows what happens during a typical menstrual cycle of 28 days. The length of the cycle will vary from woman to woman. (a) Fluctuation in the levels of the hormones oestrogen and progesterone throughout a complete menstrual cycle. (b) A follicle enlarges in the ovary and, at ovulation, ruptures to release its ovum. The remains of the follicle then form the corpus luteum. (c) The surface layer of endometrium is shed during menstruation, after which the endometrial lining of the womb builds up again as it prepares for the possible implantation of a fertilised egg. If no egg implants, the cycle starts again, with the shedding of the endometrium.

At puberty, the hypothalamus in the brain starts to produce hormones which stimulate the pituitary gland to release other hormones into the body's circulation. These pituitary hormones include **follicle-stimulating hormone** (**FSH**) and **luteinising hormone (LH)**, both of which act directly on the ovaries.

As the level of FSH increases, follicles in the ovaries start to mature and to produce the hormone **oestrogen**. The level of LH then rises to stimulate ovulation. The first follicle to mature releases its ovum and collapses, forming a corpus luteum.

Unless the released ovum is fertilised and implants in the endometrium within 7 days of ovulation, the levels of progesterone and oestrogen fall, and the endometrium cannot be maintained. Approximately 14 days after ovulation, the endometrium therefore breaks down and its blood vessels rupture: menstrual bleeding occurs. A new menstrual cycle begins as FSH is once again secreted. Menstruation can therefore be viewed as a failure of pregnancy.

Some 10–120 ml (1–12 dessertspoons) of blood are lost in each period, the average being about 50 ml. Menstruation normally occurs at intervals of 24 to 34 days (average 28 days), and the bleeding phase can last from 1 to 8 days (average 5 days). Day 1 of the menstrual cycle is the day on which bleeding starts, and the last day of the cycle is the day before the next period begins.

The menopause

Menstruation normally stops in women in Western Europe at about the age of 49 to 51. Strictly speaking, the **menopause** is the final period a woman experiences, although the term is used loosely to describe the time leading up to the last period. The **climacteric** is a more accurate term for the symptoms occurring before, during and after the final menstruation. Occasionally, a premature menopause may occur, when menstruation ceases spontaneously before the age of 40.

Hormone replacement therapy

As women approach their menopause, the decreasing levels of oestrogen are responsible for various symptoms as well as for other important changes: the bones start to become brittle as calcium is lost from them, and there is an increased risk of heart attacks and strokes. The brittle bones of **osteoporosis** can be easily broken, and complications following a broken hip are a significant cause of death in older women. Hormone replace-ment therapy (HRT) is now widely used to replace the naturally occurring hormones.

Women who have not had a hysterectomy, and those who have had an endometrial resection, can be given combined HRT – oestrogen and one of the synthetic progesterone analogues called **progestogens**. The progestogen protects the endometrial lining of the womb and therefore menstruation will continue. Oestrogen alone can be given to women who have had a hys-terectomy. The hormones are available as tablets, patches or implants.

Many women experience breast pain, fluid retention or irri-tability for a few weeks after starting HRT, but these side-effects usually settle down, and serious problems are rare. Women who have migraines while taking HRT will probably have to stop the treatment.

Studies of large numbers of women have been carried out over several years, and these suggest that the risks of HRT are small, and far outweighed by its benefits. Some doctors feel that HRT should be started some years before the menopause, as bone loss begins in a woman's 40s. The treatment can be con-tinued for the rest of a woman's life.

CHAPTER 2

Investigations and decisions

Hysterectomies are carried out to treat various disorders (see chart below), most of which become apparent as irregular or heavy periods, or as pain in the pelvis during or between the periods. The most common menstrual disorders are described in Chapter 3.

If your periods have become heavy, painful or irregular, there may be a choice of treatments available to you (see Chapter 4). Your GP may be able to discover the cause of your problem, and perhaps prescribe a drug to deal with it. If not, it may be suggested that you see a consultant for further investigations and advice.

Indications for hysterectomy. Hysterectomies performed for various conditions expressed as approximate percentages of the total number of hysterectomies carried out in the UK.

Medical condition	Percentage
Fibroids	28
Menstrual disorders	27
Cancer	10
Endometriosis	9
Prolapse	9
Benign ovarian tumours	5
Cervical pre-cancer	4
Others (e.g. Caesarean hysterectomy)	8

Visiting your GP

If you are pre-menopausal, you may have consulted your GP because your periods have changed or you may have noticed other symptoms or signs, such as continual tiredness, and your GP may discover that you are anaemic. **Anaemia** can be due to a heavy loss of blood, leading to a low level of haemoglobin, the oxygen-carrying compound present within the red blood cells.

Some women are surprised when, following careful questioning by their doctors, they are told that their periods are much heavier than average. They may have been having unusually heavy periods all their lives without realising it, and have continued to cope.

Your menstrual history

When you visit your GP you will be asked numerous questions so that a clear picture can be built up of the most likely cause of your particular problem. Your GP will want to know the date of your last menstrual period and what your menstrual cycle is like, i.e. how many days of bleeding you have and the number of days between episodes of bleeding. Before you go to see your GP, it is a good idea to keep a careful note, for a couple of months at least, of the dates on which your periods started, how many days they lasted, and any days on which you had spotting of blood. To be able to estimate how heavy your bleeding is, your GP may want to know whether you pass blood clots during your period, which look like dark pieces of liver, or experience flooding of blood which gushes out and down your legs and cannot be adequately controlled by sanitary pads or tampons.

You may also be asked if you avoid wearing white clothes during your periods; how many sanitary towels or tampons you use, and whether you need to use more than one at a time; or if your bleeding is so heavy that you avoid social functions or work or doing a large supermarket shop when it occurs.

Your GP will also want to know how your periods have changed over the years, and whether you have any bleeding between periods. This may be nothing more than some light brown spots, or it can be almost as heavy as a period itself.

Some women bleed constantly once their periods change. A typical pattern for many is increasingly heavy and more frequent periods until bleeding is continuous. You must consult your GP if this occurs.

Painful sexual intercourse

Your doctor will probably ask you if you have bleeding following sexual intercourse, and whether intercourse is painful. The pain can either be superficial, occurring at the entrance to the vagina, or can come from deep inside. This latter form of pain, called **deep dyspareunia**, may be associated with disorders of the womb, and its cause may have to be investigated further.

Your GP will also need to know when you had your last cervical smear, and is likely to do another one.

Abdominal pain

You may be asked whether you have any abdominal pain, pain associated with periods, or any urinary or bowel symptoms, such as frequency or incontinence. If it is necessary for you to have a hysterectomy, it might be possible for something to be done about symptoms of this sort at the same time.

Contraceptive history

It will be helpful if you can give your GP details of your contraceptive history. Although these should be available on your medical records, if you have been going to a different doctor or family planning clinic for contraceptive advice, your GP may not know about it.

Periods get heavier once the contraceptive pill is stopped. So, for instance, a woman who has been taking the pill for some years and then decides to be sterilised in her 30s may find that after sterilisation her periods become much heavier. This may be because they were artificially light when she was taking the pill.

The intra-uterine contraceptive device (IUCD) known as the coil can make periods heavy, painful and possibly irregular. If you have an IUCD and get these symptoms, your GP is likely to recommend that it is removed. The contraceptives Depo-provera and Norplant can also cause irregular bleeding, but not usually heavy bleeding. **Depo-provera** is a long-acting synthetic hormone given in the form of an injection, the effects of which last for 3 months. **Norplant** is a contraceptive drug contained in a matchstick-sized implant which is inserted under the skin, usually in the arm, and continues to be effective for about 5 years. Once the implant has been removed, fertility usually returns within a few days.

Obstetric history

To complete the picture, your GP will review your obstetric history, asking how many children you have had and how they were born. More importantly for women of child-bearing age, the GP will discuss with them their plans for a family.

A woman in her 30s who is experiencing problems with her periods should certainly have had careful discussions with her partner, at least before she sees a consultant, as obviously hysterectomy and similar treatments preclude her having more children.

Physical examination

Your GP will normally examine your abdomen, feeling for swellings and tenderness, and will then carry out an internal vaginal examination. This is known as a **bimanual examination**, and involves feeling the cervix with one or two fingers inserted through the vagina. At the same time, the doctor presses with the other hand on the lower abdomen to try to feel the top end of the uterus. This allows the doctor to assess the size, shape,

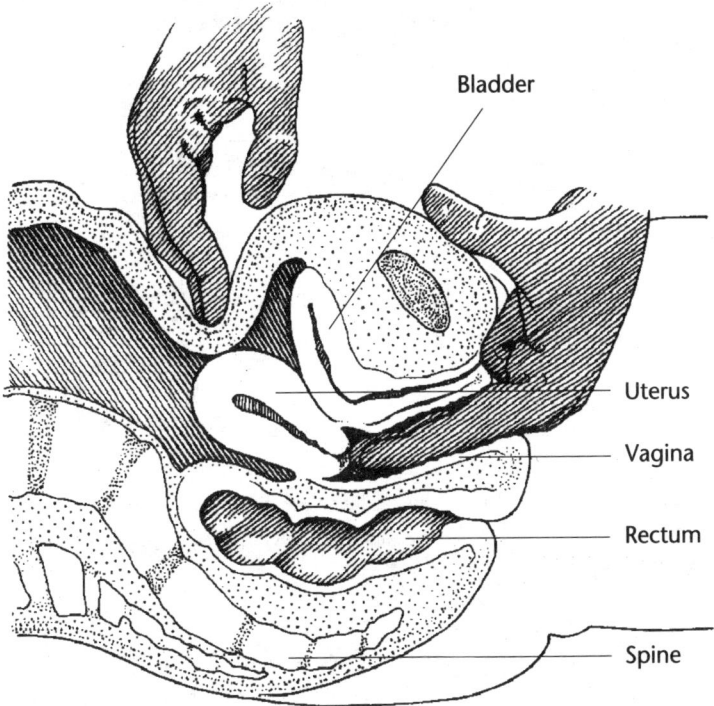

Bimanual examination. The doctor inserts two fingers into the vagina to touch the cervix. With the other hand pressing on the abdomen, the top of the uterus may be felt, and an idea obtained of how large and mobile it is.

mobility and position of the uterus. The ovaries may also be felt if they are enlarged.

Following this, another examination may be done with an instrument called a **speculum**. The metal or plastic speculum is lubricated and inserted into the vagina, the walls of which can thus be parted to allow the doctor to see the cervix.

The vaginal examination is uncomfortable but should not be painful. If it is painful, do tell your doctor.

It is quite possible to be examined during a period. Although

This part of the speculum is closed and inserted into the vagina

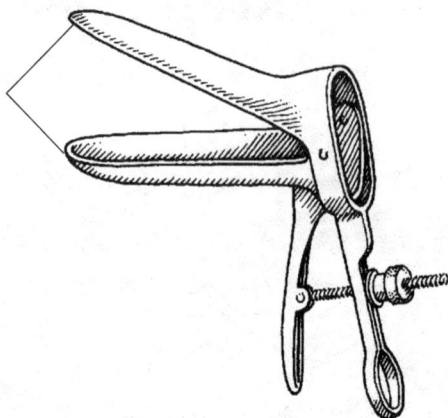

A speculum. The blades of the speculum are closed and inserted into the vagina. The blades are then opened as much as is possible without causing undue discomfort. The walls of the vagina are thus separated, allowing the doctor a clear view of the cervix.

many women find it embarrassing, it is important that you are examined and GPs are used to doing it. However, if you really cannot face the prospect, do phone your GP to cancel your appointment and to make another at a later date when your period is finished. However, if your period does not stop, do not wait to see your doctor. It is important in this situation that you overcome your embarrassment and are examined.

Cervical smear

Most doctors will do a cervical smear if a woman complains of irregular bleeding. Again, this may be an uncomfortable but not a painful procedure. A speculum is inserted into the vagina so that the cervix can be seen, and a specially shaped wooden spatula is gently rotated against the skin at the lower end of the cervix to remove a small sample of cells. The cells are then spread onto a microscopy slide, fixed with a chemical, and sent

to the laboratory for cytological examination under a microscope.

Once the doctor has completed the examinations, you may be
offered medication, or may be referred to a consultant in gynaecology. If you would prefer to see a gynaecologist who is a
woman, you should ask your GP if this can be arranged.

Visiting the consultant

{A **gynaecologist** is a doctor who specialises in the diagnosis
and treatment of diseases affecting the female genital organs.
An **obstetrician** cares for women during pregnancy, childbirth
and the period immediately after childbirth. However, in the UK,
99% of doctors working in these fields specialise in both gynaecology and obstetrics.}

Once your GP has written to a consultant asking for an appointment to be made for you, you may have to wait anything from a
few weeks to several months.

The consultant will ask you questions similar to those your
GP asked, and may also assess your general state of health, asking about your past medical history, any medication you are taking, your smoking habits and social life. Unlike many other types
of surgery, the decision to do a hysterectomy or similar operation does involve consideration of a woman's personal circumstances, for example whether she is sexually active, has
completed her family, and whether, if she has a regular partner
or husband, he is likely to support her in her decision and after
her operation.

Consultants often see women in their 20s who find their
periods inconvenient, have no children, are not in permanent
relationships, and want a hysterectomy. The consultant may not
agree to this request, as to undertake a major and irreversible
operation in these circumstances may not be in the woman's

15

best interests: she may change her mind in the future if her circumstances change.

The consultant will examine you thoroughly, as described above. You will probably be given a bimanual examination, a speculum examination, and possibly a cervical smear. There are various other tests your consultant may want to arrange (see below), and an appointment may be made for you to enter hospital for these to be carried out if they cannot be done at the out-patients' clinic.

Endometrial biopsy

If your bleeding has been irregular, the consultant may suggest doing an endometrial biopsy. Endometrial biopsy is the alternative to dilatation and curettage (D & C), and is carried out to exclude endometrial cancer, particularly for women over the age of 35. Endometrial cancer is extremely rare in women below this age, and is therefore not usually looked for. Although it is statistically unlikely that if you have irregular bleeding you will have cancer, endometrial cancer is curable if discovered early.

For women in their 40s whose periods are heavy but regular, endometrial biopsy may not be necessary.

The consultant will use a small plastic tube to remove endometrial tissue from the lining of the uterus. Unlike a D & C, endometrial biopsy does not involve dilatation of the cervix, and the tube can be slipped through the cervix with minimum discomfort to obtain a sample of the endometrium. No anaesthetic is required.

Normally, the consultant will also use a speculum to look at the cervix and may possibly take a smear.

Dilatation and curettage

Although some consultants still do D & Cs, this operation is less common than it was a few years ago. It is a diagnostic procedure, with no long-term treatment element. The first period after a D & C may be lighter, but the second is usually almost back to normal, or even heavier, and the third one is back to normal.

As dilatation of the cervix is a painful procedure, the operation is usually carried out using a general anaesthetic. Metal probes or dilators of increasing diameter are first inserted into the cervical canal to stretch it. A small spoon-shaped instrument called a curette is then introduced into the uterus, and its sharp edge is used to scrape a sample of tissue from the endometrium. The tissue is then examined under a microscope to detect any abnormality.

Hysteroscopy and biopsy

Some consultants prefer to do a hysteroscopy and biopsy rather than an endometrial biopsy. This is sometimes done under general anaesthetic and sometimes under local anaesthetic, depending in part on the facilities available and on the woman concerned. For example, for an elderly and nervous woman who has not had any children, general anaesthetic may be recommended. Most consultants will take into account any anaesthetic preference stated by the woman herself.

Hysteroscopy involves inserting a small telescope (approximately the diameter of a pencil) into the uterus and actually looking into the cavity for any swellings such as fibroids (see p. 24) or polyps. A **polyp** is a small swelling on the end of a stalk which may not be detected during endometrial biopsy. There is, however, no evidence to show that hysteroscopy is more likely than endometrial biopsy to pick up cancer, and it is therefore not often used routinely.

Hysteroscopy is usually accompanied by a biopsy. A sample of endometrium is obtained by any of the methods described above, and is put into formalin to preserve the cells for examination by a pathologist. It may be possible to tell from this sample at what stage of the menstrual cycle the woman is and whether she is ovulating – but that is not the reason for this biopsy.

The biopsy is the most important part of the procedure because it may not always be possible to see an early cancer, particularly in a woman who is bleeding heavily.

Ultrasound scan

An ultrasound scan may be done if the consultant was not able to feel your uterus or needs more information about its size or shape or the thickness of the endometrium. It involves passing high-frequency sound waves into the body, and is the same process as that used for fetal scanning in pregnant women. When the sound waves meet a solid object within the body cavity, they are reflected back like an echo. A computer processes the waves and builds up a picture which is displayed on a screen and interpreted by someone trained in ultrasonography.

A pelvic ultrasound examination can be abdominal or vaginal. For an abdominal scan, a special jelly-like substance is smeared onto the abdomen, and a probe is gently moved over it. This is not a painful procedure, but it is necessary to have a full bladder while it is carried out and this can cause some discomfort.

The vaginal scan is done by inserting a small probe, about the size of one or two fingers, gently into the vagina. The process is painless.

Blood tests

The only other investigation that the consultant is likely to require is a blood test to detect anaemia. Many women become anaemic without being aware of it, and the presence of anaemia needs to be known about before any operation is undertaken. If you are found to be anaemic, you will probably be treated with iron, in the form of tablets or occasionally injections. When bleeding has been very heavy, blood transfusion may be necessary.

Occasionally, blood coagulation disorders or thyroid disease can cause problems with periods, and a blood test may be arranged to test thyroid function and the ability of the blood to form clots.

Discussion with the consultant

After taking your history, doing the examination and tests, the consultant will discuss with you your treatment options (see Chapter 4). You should not feel hurried into making an instant decision about what to do. If your consultant does not give you the chance to think things through, you can always ask for time to consider what has been said and then to come back. In fact, it is most important that you think things through carefully and, if you have a partner, discuss your options with him.

Because of the many treatments that are available, it is better not to attend the out-patients' clinic with set ideas, such as, for example, that you want a hysterectomy. It is better to listen to what the treatment options are and to take time to make your decision.

Examination by medical students

You may be asked if a medical student can examine you at the out-patients' clinic or while you are under anaesthetic just before your operation begins. Only one student is permitted to do a vaginal examination on a patient who is under anaesthetic, and the woman's consent is always obtained beforehand, either in writing or verbally, depending on the hospital's policy. The student will perform a vaginal examination and possibly also a speculum examination.

It is very important that medical students are able to do these examinations, both on women who are awake and on those who are anaesthetised, and it is less embarrassing for both the woman and the student if done while she is anaesthetised. It is also easier for the student to learn if the examination is carried out when the woman's muscles are relaxed.

If you are being treated in a teaching hospital, you are virtually certain to be asked; you may be approached if you are in a district hospital which is attended by medical students.

However, you can, of course, refuse your permission if you prefer; the decision is yours entirely and will not affect your treatment in any way.

Making a decision

Unless a woman has uterine cancer, there is never any absolute necessity for her to have a hysterectomy. To do so has to be her own decision, depending on how much her periods are affecting her life.

It may be wise to accept surgical treatment if for 1 or 2 days every month you are unable to leave the house, if you have to plan your holidays around your periods, are losing time off work, or if drug treatment has proved ineffective (see p. 29). The affect that heavy periods have on a woman may depend on her age. If you are in your 30s and have to spend 2 days in the house every month, you will obviously want something done. If, however, you are 49 and can expect to go through the menopause within the next year or so, it may be worth putting up with it until then. Obviously, when you are 45, it is a more difficult decision.

When considering the treatment options, the overriding consideration, apart from age, is whether you have completed your family. If you do want more children, or this is possible, you can either do nothing or take medication.

The other category of women who are wise to have something done are those who are recurrently anaemic with their periods, leading to chronic ill-health. The quality of life for these women is much improved by an operation.

There are old-style gynaecologists who believe that if a woman is not anaemic she cannot be having heavy periods and is making a fuss. Most doctors, however, do not believe this anymore. Routine full blood counts which are done to measure the level of haemoglobin in the blood are not an accurate way of estimating a woman's iron stores. A more accurate method is to measure the ferritin, as this can be very low even when the haemoglobin is normal.

If you feel your periods are restricting your life, however heavy or light they might be, and that treatment is more desirable than putting up with them, most gynaecologists will be happy to treat you.

There is an interesting new category of women seeking treatment: post-menopausal women on hormone replacement therapy. The old-fashioned view would have been that the HRT must be stopped and the problem will go away. But HRT now has such proven benefits that many gynaecologists will be happy to treat women in this category for their periods. Usually medication is all that is required, including altering the hormone dose or possibly changing to another type. If this is not sufficient, an endometrial resection can be considered (see p. 74). It is unlikely a hysterectomy will be necessary.

There are various factors you should take into account when considering having any type of hysterectomy. Following an abdominal or vaginal hysterectomy (see pp. 66–71), you may be in hospital for up to a week – the average time being about 5 to 6 days. When you go home you may not be able immediately to lift children, and may therefore need help with childcare and housework.

It is common to have up to 3 months off work after a hysterectomy, although some self-employed or well-motivated women whose jobs do not involve heavy lifting go back to work after 6 weeks or less.

A hysterectomy is not a simple operation; it is a major operation which is normally carried out without any serious complications. However, complications can arise and these need to be borne in mind (see Chapter 11).

For women who have had regular, normal cervical smears, there is no need to have further smears after hysterectomy, although those with a history of cervical abnormalities may be well advised to continue to have regular cervical smears – for how long depends on the particular abnormality. As the cervix is still in place following an endometrial resection, cervical smears will continue to be necessary.

If you need a translator

Women who have a limited understanding of English, or who do not speak the language well, should take with them, to all appointments with their GP or consultant, a *woman* who can translate for them. Some women visit their doctors with their young sons, to act as translators, but this is inappropriate when discussing matters about which the boys have almost no understanding. There have been cases where women who do not speak English have undergone hysterectomies and then returned later to their doctors to complain that they are unable to conceive. It is important that women know exactly what any proposed treatment involves before they agree to it.

CHAPTER 3

Common menstrual disorders

Menstrual disorders can be due to a variety of conditions, and some of the more common ones are explained in this chapter.

Bleeding between periods, known as **intermenstrual bleeding**, or after the menopause, **post-menopausal bleeding**, is usually due to a benign condition, but it can be a sign of cancer of the uterus or cervix and should therefore be investigated.

Amenorrhoea

This is the complete absence of bleeding. It can be primary, if bleeding has never occurred, or secondary, if bleeding stops following a previously normal menstrual pattern. It is, however, a normal symptom of pregnancy – its most common cause.

Dysmenorrhoea

This is the term given to pain occurring during menstruation. Again, it may be primary, if it has no associated problems, or secondary, if it occurs with disease or infection.

Dysfunctional uterine bleeding

If the balance of the hormones oestrogen and progesterone is disturbed for some reason, the periods may become heavy or irregular. Dysfunctional uterine bleeding is the term used for irregular or heavy bleeding for which no cause can be found. Although hormone tablets will usually correct a hormone imbalance, a persistent problem can be treated by surgery, such as a hysterectomy.

Dysfunctional uterine bleeding can occur in various forms.

- **Menorrhagia** describes a normal menstrual cycle with heavy blood loss, or an increased number of days of heavy but regular bleeding.

- **Epimenorrhoea** and **polymenorrhoea** are terms used to describe a condition in which there is normal menstruation which occurs too often.

- **Threshold bleeding** occurs as a result of fluctuating low levels of oestrogen and an absence of progesterone. It is most common at the time of the menarche and at the menopause.

Fibroids

Fibroids are muscular swellings within the muscular outer layer of myometrium in the womb which, particularly if they are large, can cause heavy bleeding. A lump may be felt in the lower abdomen, or there may be pressure on the bladder or bowel causing increased frequency. Sometimes a hysterectomy is necessary if heavy bleeding or bladder or bowel symptoms are troublesome. Fibroids will normally shrink after the menopause, but do not always do so.

Prolapse of the womb

As women get older, the ligaments and muscles which hold the womb in place within the body cavity may weaken, allowing the womb to drop down into the vagina. In severe cases, the womb

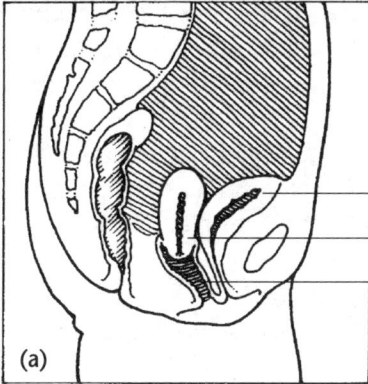

Bladder
Uterus
Vagina

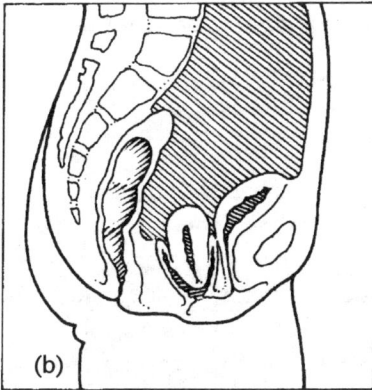

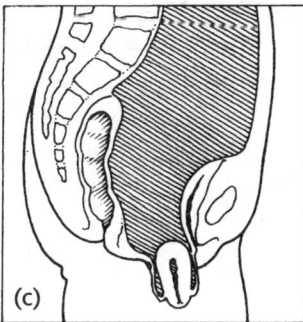

Prolapse of the womb. (a) The womb is starting to push down into the top of the vagina. (b) The prolapse has worsened, and the womb has entered the vaginal canal. (c) The womb has now prolapsed so far that it is starting to protrude through the external vaginal opening. Pressure is also being exerted on the bladder as the walls of the vagina collapse.

can protrude through the vagina and be visible outside the body. Prolapse of the womb can also occur following childbirth, or when another stress, such as chronic constipation, weakens its support.

The first symptom of a prolapsed womb may be stress incontinence, with urine escaping during sneezing or coughing. The bowel may be affected, leading to constipation. Sometimes, standing for long periods can cause discomfort and a feeling of heaviness in the vagina.

A hysterectomy to remove the womb will usually relieve these symptoms. However, you should ask your consultant how likely it is that your bladder or bowel symptoms will be improved by hysterectomy, or whether another form of treatment will be necessary as well.

Endometriosis

Normally, during a period, the blood shed with the endometrial lining of the womb escapes down the cervix and out through the vagina. In some women, for unexplained reasons, seed-like endometrial cells occur outside the uterus, most commonly on the outer surface of the uterus or on the ovaries, bladder or bowel. These 'seedlings' of endometrium start to grow outside the womb, and are subject to the same hormonal influences as the endometrium itself. They therefore bleed as normal during each period, but the blood is unable to escape. As blood builds up, it causes pain and can result in organs sticking together. These **adhesions** can make conception difficult.

Treatment with drugs may be successful, but for women who do not want to have any more children, removal of the womb and both ovaries is an option.

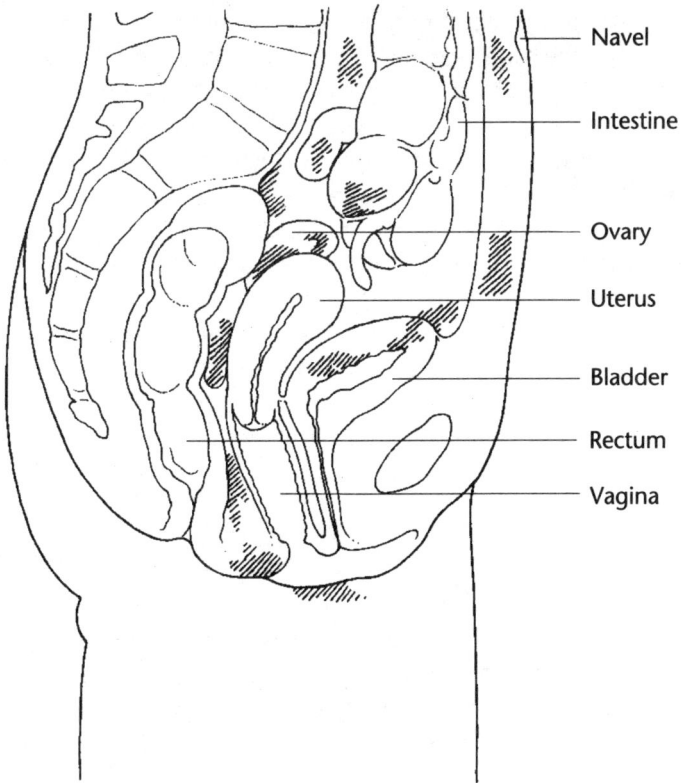

Endometriosis. This diagram shows the sites at which endometriosis (shaded areas) can occur in the pelvic and abdominal cavities.

Cancer of the genital organs

In Britain, women are offered regular cervical smears to try to detect abnormalities which may develop into cancer of the neck of the womb – **cervical cancer**. Regular smears are important so that any **pre-cancerous** changes in the cells of the cervix can be detected. Not all women with pre-cancerous cell changes will go on to develop cervical cancer, but they are at risk, and therefore have much to gain from early treatment. Pre-cancer can be treated by the surgical removal of a small piece of the cervix and this is unlikely to have any adverse effect on the periods, fertility or pregnancy. Established cervical cancer requires the removal of the uterus by Wertheim's hysterectomy (see p. 36) or radio-therapy.

Irregular bleeding can be an early sign of cervical cancer or of **endometrial cancer** – cancer of the lining of the womb. For endometrial cancer, a hysterectomy will be necessary. Spread of this type of cancer does not occur at an early stage, and there-fore, if detected soon enough, the chances of cure are good.

Cancer of the ovaries is more difficult to detect, particularly during its early stages. The uterus and both ovaries will usually have to be removed if this is present.

Ovarian cysts

A cyst is a fluid-filled swelling which can occur almost anywhere in the body. Normal ovaries contain small cysts (follicles), vary-ing in size from a pinhead to a pea. Every month one follicular cyst enlarges to 2 to 3 cm prior to ovulation. Ovarian cysts larger than 6 cm (about 2 inches) will need to be investigated as they may be other than enlarged cysts. They normally require treatment, involving the removal either of the cyst itself, in an operation called a **cystectomy**, or of the affected ovary by oophorectomy.

CHAPTER 4

Treatment options

Not all of the treatment options available are suitable for every woman, and you will have to be guided in the choice of treatment by your consultant. If you have heavy periods, you will have to make your own decision as to whether to have a hysterectomy, but if your surgeon says you are not suitable for a vaginal hysterectomy – which will usually be because your uterus is too big – and the operation can only be done by the abdominal route, you must accept this. If you are particularly anxious, you can always ask for a second opinion; your GP will be able to arrange for you to see another consultant.

DRUG OPTIONS

There are several groups of drugs available for treating menstrual problems. The basic types are as follows.

1   **Non-steroidal anti-inflammatory drugs (NSAIDs)**, e.g. ibuprofen (Brufen), and mefenamic acid (Ponstan Forte). Some NSAIDs can be bought over the counter at pharmacies. They are painkillers which help relieve period pains, but they also have an anti-inflammatory action. The NSAIDs have been proved in studies to decrease heavy bleeding significantly. Their great advantage is that they need only be taken during the time of menstrual bleeding, and they are therefore the first line of treatment for women who wish to conceive.

2 **Anti-fibrinolytics**, e.g. ethamsylate (Dicynene), and tranexamic acid (Cyklokapron). These also only need to be taken during menstruation, but may be more effective if continued for 2 weeks. Their actions are complicated but they have been proved to decrease bleeding. They are slightly more expensive than the NSAIDs and have no effect on pain. But, again, they can be used by women who wish to conceive.

3 **Oral contraceptives**. For women who are not trying to conceive, the safest and most effective drug is the oral contraceptive pill, of which there are several different types available. Paradoxically, this can cause or cure irregular bleeding. For women who do not smoke, it is now possible to take a form of the oral contraceptive pill right through to the menopause. The doses being used are much lower than they were in the 1960s and 1970s, and they are correspondingly safer. For teenagers who have heavy periods, the oral contraceptive pill may be the first choice. However, if there is some reason not to take it, progestogens can be used.

Once the drugs are stopped, conception can occur, although there may be a short delay.

4 **Progestogens**. A progestogen is a synthetic drug which mimics the action of the naturally occurring hormone progesterone. The role of progesterone in the body is to prepare the lining of the uterus for an expected pregnancy. It also causes breast engorgement and fluid retention. The synthetic drugs are used in the form of oral progestogens, e.g. norethisterone, medroxy-progesterone acetate. As with any drugs, there are side-effects associated with them, and these will be listed on the container. They may cause weight gain, mood changes and **oedema** – swelling of the lower abdomen, fingers, hands and ankles, which is due to fluid retention.

Although progestogens have not been proved to decrease the amount of bleeding, some women find them effective. They seem to act by regularising the cycle, and a large enough dose will stop bleeding. However, large doses cannot be given on a long-term basis. Irregular menstrual cycles can normally be controlled by small doses taken on a cyclical basis, usually for 1 to 3 weeks in each cycle. They are probably most effective for use by teenagers or older women.

Progestogens can also be given in the form of Depo-provera or Norplant implants (see p. 12). Although the implants do decrease heavy bleeding, they tend to cause irregular bleeding. Norplant has an advantage over drugs given in the form of an injection and which, once injected cannot be taken out, as the implant can be removed if necessary.

Another exciting development in this field has been the progestogen-containing IUCDs. Although IUCDs are normally associated with heavy periods, this new type contains a progestogen, acts as a contraceptive, and decreases bleeding. These IUCDs may be widely used in the future and may be worth a try, for example before proceeding to an endometrial resection or a hysterectomy. They can, however, cause irregular spotting of blood which some women find intolerable. Their advantage is that because the progestogen is given locally in the uterus, a lower dose can be used and fewer side-effects seem to occur.

5   **Danazol**. If treatment with progestogen fails, danazol may be prescribed. This is a synthetic hormone which is commercially available as Danol. Its use is recommended for only 6 months as it can produce changes in cholesterol levels and liver function. If given in high enough doses, it

will reduce the amount of bleeding. However, danazol is androgenic, and can lead to the development of male characteristics such as facial hair (**hirsutism**), oily or spotty skin, and deepening of the voice. Women are often not happy with the doses required to control their periods: although 200 mg a day may decrease the heaviness of the periods, some women require up to 800 mg a day. At this level, the side-effects are often intolerable.

6 **Luteinising-hormone releasing hormone analogues (LHRH)**, e.g. goserelin. Goserelin is given as an injection, once a month. There are some other LHRH analogues which can be inhaled, but these may need to be taken several times a day, and can be less convenient.

The drugs in this group stop the periods completely and induce a temporary menopause, with all the symptoms of menopause such as hot flushes and night sweats. The drugs are extremely effective and will stop the periods within 2 months. Because of the risks of osteoporosis, which causes the bones to become brittle, it is not advisable to continue taking these drugs for longer than 6 months.

The LHRH analogues are not used routinely to treat heavy periods. They are normally only used for young women who have extremely heavy periods and fibroids but who want to conceive. The drugs can shrink fibroids and control the periods, possibly allowing conception to occur.

SURGICAL OPTIONS

Myomectomy

Drugs in the LHRH analogue group may also be given to women to shrink their fibroids prior to surgery, making them easier and safer to remove. The effect is temporary, and the fibroids will start to regrow within 6 to 12 months.

Fibroids can be removed surgically by **myomectomy**. They are simply cut out of the uterus, leaving the uterus itself in place. This operation is not common, and is only ever performed for women who wish to have children. It is a difficult operation and has significantly more associated risk than does a hysterectomy. It may make subsequent hysterectomy more difficult, and it is therefore not a suitable option for a woman who has completed her family but would simply like to control her periods.

Hysterectomy

There are three types of hysterectomy which can be performed: abdominal, vaginal and laparoscopic. Abdominal and vaginal hysterectomies take about an hour; the laparoscopic operation takes rather longer, but the stay in hospital is shorter. Full details of these operations are given in Chapter 7.

Abdominal hysterectomy

Abdominal hysterectomy usually involves a transverse cut in the abdomen just under the pubic hairline. This is known as a 'bikini' incision as it would be hidden by the bottom half of a bikini. Occasionally the operation may require a midline, vertical incision if the uterus is very enlarged. The uterus, with or without the ovaries, can be removed by this method.

Because abdominal hysterectomy requires an incision in the abdomen, it is slightly more painful post-operatively than the other types of surgery. Coughing tends to be avoided as it can be painful, and therefore chest infections can be more likely. As mobilisation is delayed following an abdominal hysterectomy, there may also be more risk of blood clots developing in the legs (**deep vein thrombosis**, DVT) and breaking off and travelling in the bloodstream to the lungs (**pulmonary embolism**).

(See p. 51 for a more detailed explanation.) Injections of heparin (see p. 52) are therefore often given routinely.

The operation does have the advantage of allowing the abdominal cavity to be inspected and the ovaries to be removed, if necessary.

Sexual intercourse following an abdominal hysterectomy should not be significantly affected. The vagina will end blindly, rather than in the cervix, but it should be of the same length and capacity. Having said that, sexual intercourse following hysterectomy has never been properly evaluated, and some women find that their sexual pleasure is diminished when their cervix has been removed.

Vaginal hysterectomy

Vaginal hysterectomy involves removing the whole uterus and cervix through the vagina. (This is not the suction method – there is no suction involved.) The vaginal walls are retracted and the uterus is pulled down and cut out. The operation is basically the same as an abdominal hysterectomy but there is no abdominal incision.

A vaginal hysterectomy is probably preferable if it is an option, particularly for women whose cervical smears have been abnormal. The surgeon has to decide whether the uterus is small enough and mobile enough to be removed this way. If a woman has had previous surgery (including caesarean section), endometriosis or infection, her uterus may have become fixed inside the abdomen and may not descend, and vaginal hysterectomy will therefore not be possible.

It is not usually possible to remove the ovaries or inspect them in detail with this method, although they may be felt for the presence of a tumour. Vaginal hysterectomy is not suitable for women who have ovarian cysts.

The surgeon may decide to assess which method is possible at the time of operation, or may do an examination and D & C (see p. 16) with the woman under anaesthetic.

A vaginal hysterectomy is the method of choice to remove a uterus which has already prolapsed into the vagina. It is also possible to repair any prolapse of the vaginal wall at the same time (see p. 24). Having a hysterectomy does not preclude the possibility of a prolapse developing in later life, as it is the anterior and posterior walls of the *vagina* which often prolapse, rather than the uterus itself.

The recovery following vaginal hysterectomy is less painful and may be slightly shorter than after the abdominal operation, although not significantly so.

Laparoscopically assisted hysterectomy

Laparoscopic hysterectomy is newly available in some centres in the UK, the commonly used form being laparoscopically assisted vaginal hysterectomy. As this operation takes longer to perform than a conventional hysterectomy, many surgeons are reluctant to do it – not only because the period of anaesthesia is longer, but also because fewer operations can be carried out.

An instrument called a **laparoscope** is inserted into the abdominal cavity through a small incision, and other surgical instruments are introduced through two similar incisions.

The operation involves dividing the ovarian and uterine blood supplies using automatic clamps. If necessary, the ovaries may also be removed at the same time. The bladder is pushed down from above, and the operation is then completed vaginally.

This operation may be suitable for women who cannot have a vaginal hysterectomy, perhaps because they have a large or fixed uterus.

Laparoscopically assisted vaginal hysterectomy is not done as day-case surgery because it involves cutting major blood vessels, and therefore a risk of bleeding in the first 24 hours postoperatively. However, it is often possible to go home the day after surgery, and the recovery period is usually shorter than for other types of hysterectomy.

If the operation is found to be technically impossible once surgery begins, the surgeon may have to convert to a traditional abdominal hysterectomy. This must be borne in mind before you choose this option.

Sub-total hysterectomy

In this operation, the body of the uterus is removed, leaving the cervix behind. As there is no endometrium in the cervix, the periods will cease.

Sub-total hysterectomy was popular many years ago but fell into disrepute because if cervical cancer does develop subsequently, it can spread quickly and is difficult to treat. It therefore began to be done only if it was technically impossible to remove the cervix. However, sub-total hysterectomy may become more popular in the future as the disadvantages of the cervix being left in place are now minimal due to the improved quality of cervical smears and the treatment available if pre-cancerous changes are detected. Retaining the cervix may result in less damage to the nerves that are important in urinary and sexual function.

As the cervix remains in place, sub-total hysterectomy cannot be done via the vaginal route, and is therefore done abdominally or laparoscopically.

Wertheim's hysterectomy

Also known as a **radical hysterectomy,** this operation is rare, and is only carried out in an attempt to effect a complete cure for cancer of the cervix which has been detected at an early stage of development.

Wertheim's hysterectomy involves the removal of the uterus, both ovaries, the top third of the vagina, the tissue in the broad ligament (known as the parametrium), and all the pelvic lymph nodes. It also involves extensive separation of the bladder and the ureters (which carry urine from the kidneys to the bladder) from the surrounding tissue. Damage to the bladder and ureters is therefore more of a risk with this type of operation than during the less radical forms of hysterectomy. Blood transfusion is more likely to be required during a Wertheim's hysterectomy, and radiotherapy may be necessary following it.

As this is a serious and difficult operation to perform, it must be done by a specialist in gynaecological cancer who has specific experience with this type of surgery. There are normally only one or two such specialists in each health region, and it may therefore be necessary to travel to a hospital outside your immediate area if you need to have this operation.

As a Wertheim's hysterectomy is a radical and relatively uncommon operation, it is not dealt with in detail in this book. It does require a longer stay in hospital than any of the other types of hysterectomy, and you will be given specific advice and information if you are to undergo this operation.

Oophorectomy

If the ovaries are removed at the same time as an abdominal hysterectomy is done, this will induce an artificial menopause, and it is advisable to have hormone replacement therapy, at least until the age of 50. Many women find that they immediately feel better when HRT is started (see p. 8), and that they experience an increase in their energy levels and feelings of well-being. Removing the ovaries and starting HRT may also help relieve the symptoms of pre-menstrual tension.

It may be considered that, generally, women who are post-menopausal or who are approaching the menopause have nothing to gain by keeping their ovaries as they will soon cease to function and HRT will be needed. Removal of the ovaries also, of course, removes any risk of ovarian cancer. For women who are under 40, and who do not have any disease of the ovaries, and especially for those who do not like the prospect of taking tablets, the ovaries should be retained if possible, otherwise HRT may be required for many years. Between the ages of 40 and 50, the decision to have the ovaries removed is a personal one, to be made by individual women in consultation with their surgeons.

Women whose ovaries are diseased in any way, who have endometriosis (see p. 26) or cysts, should have their ovaries removed at the time of hysterectomy. A family history of ovarian cancer may also affect the decision.

Transcervical resection of the endometrium

This is a relatively new operation which has only been under-taken in the UK since about 1988. It involves removing the endometrial lining of the uterus, leaving the uterus itself in place. The cervix is dilated, and a resectoscope (see p. 74) and an irrigating system are introduced. The surgeon can then see to cut or burn away the endometrium and the inner third of the myometrium. As the operation does not involve any incisions, and therefore there are no post-operative wounds, there is very little pain associated with it – no more than a period pain. It can therefore be performed as a day case.

Having an endometrial resection does not guarantee that the periods will stop. Figures vary from surgeon to surgeon, but, on average, the periods of about 50% of women stop or virtually stop after the operation; 40% of women still have periods, but these are less heavy; 10% of women will require either a further endometrial resection or hysterectomy, probably within 2 years. The operation is, however, worth trying in many cases as it involves just 1 day in hospital and about 7 to 14 days off work.

Before having an endometrial resection, it may be advisable to take drugs to thin the endometrium, as the thinner it is, the more likely the operation is to be successful. The drugs used are either danazol or LHRH agonists, or occasionally high-dose progestogens. They will have to be taken for 3 months pre-operatively. Most women do not seem to mind taking medication when they know it is going to lead to an operation which may relieve their menstrual problems.

The alternative to drug treatment is to do the operation immediately after a period, but this is often difficult to arrange for operations done in the National Health Service (NHS). Also, timing the operation against the menstrual cycle is probably less effective than taking medication.

As already mentioned, the periods may continue following the operation and, as the ovaries are not removed, it is still possible to conceive, although unlikely. Therefore some form of contraception is necessary because if conception does occur after endometrial resection, the placenta can implant in an abnormal way and this may be dangerous for the woman and her baby.

Because some small pockets of endometrium are almost certain to have been left behind during an endometrial resection, women are advised that when the time comes to take HRT, it should be in the form of combined oestrogen and progestogens. Progestogens are the part of the HRT that women do not like taking as they tend to be associated with bloating, depression and pre-menstrual symptoms. However, although oestrogen is effective at preventing all the symptoms of the menopause, if taken on its own when the uterus is still in place, it may cause cancer of any remaining endometrium. It can be taken alone following hysterectomy as the entire endometrium will have been removed.

Bleeding and discharge will occur after endometrial resection, normally for a few days like a period, but possibly continuing for 4 to 6 weeks. By 3 to 4 months after the operation, most women will have settled into a pattern of no bleeding or lighter, regular periods.

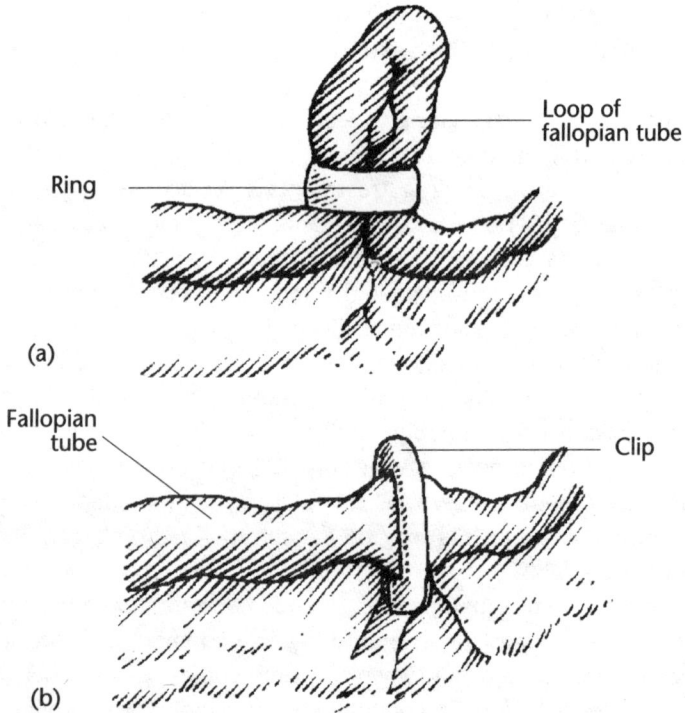

Female sterilisation. To prevent fertilisation of ova occurring within the fallopian tubes, a ring (a) or clip (b) is placed around each tube to close it off.

Laparoscopic sterilisation

It is possible for laparoscopic sterilisation to be done at the same time as an endometrial resection, and you should ask your consultant about this if appropriate. **The operation alone does not have any effect on the periods**.

Laparoscopic sterilisation usually involves placing clips or rings across the fallopian tubes to close them and prevent fertilisation of an ovum taking place within them. In some cases, if sterilisation is done after a caesarean section, the fallopian tubes are actually cut and tied off.

CHAPTER 5

Going in to hospital

You will probably receive a letter from the hospital telling you the date of your operation and any other details you need to know. Many hospitals also send out leaflets explaining the admission procedures and advising you what to take in with you. You may have been put on a shortlist so that if an unexpected gap occurs in the operating schedule, you will be asked to come in at short notice – possibly within a day or two.

Some hospitals also run **pre-admission clerking clinics** which take place anything from 2 days to a week before you are admitted for your operation. If this is the case, your admission letter will explain the procedure to you and give you the date and time of the appointment which has been arranged for you. During this clinic, a doctor will explain the operation and will answer any questions you may have. You will probably also be asked to sign a consent form to say that you have understood what is to take place (see p. 54). Any pre-operative tests that are necessary, such as a blood test, may also be done at this time so that the results can be obtained before you enter hospital for surgery.

Length of stay in hospital

The length of your stay in hospital will depend largely on what type of operation you are having. You will probably be able to go home 1 or 2 days after an endometrial resection, 3 to 5 days after a vaginal hysterectomy, and 5 to 7 days after a total abdominal hysterectomy. The more major procedure of a

Wertheim's hysterectomy will probably involve a slightly longer stay.

Day-case surgery

If you are having an endometrial resection and are otherwise fit and healthy, the consultant may have suggested at your outpatients' appointment that you be treated as a day case. Day-case surgery is, of course, not suitable for women having hysterectomies of any sort.

The average cost of an operation involving an overnight stay in hospital is approximately three to four times greater than the cost of the operation done as a day case. Now that hospital expenditure is a major consideration, day-case surgery is seen as a sensible way of cutting costs and reducing the length of waiting lists. It will be even more common when the Government's proposed reduction in the number of hospital beds comes into effect.

If you are to be treated as a day-case patient, you will be admitted to hospital an hour or two before your operation and will leave again a few hours after you have recovered from the anaesthetic. Patients have to be screened very carefully to make sure that only those whose general health is good are selected for this type of care. Women over the age of 50 are usually considered to be unsuitable for day-case surgery as health problems are more common in this age group, and therefore pre-operative tests such as chest X-rays and electrocardiograms (ECGs) may be needed. These tests can sometimes be done by a GP a week or two before the operation so that the time in hospital is kept to a minimum. Alternatively, the tests may be carried out at a pre-admission clerking clinic (see above) so that your medical history, examination and investigation results can be collated by a hospital doctor.

What to take into hospital

As you are unlikely to be in hospital for longer than a few days, you will not need to take much in with you. The following list may be helpful.

1 *Sanitary pads.* Although the hospital will probably supply sanitary pads for the first few days after your operation, you may prefer to use your own. You may be given sterile pads immediately after your operation, but can soon revert to ordinary sanitary pads. Sanitary pads are expensive, and therefore women are usually encouraged to supply their own whenever possible. Those issued by hospitals are likely to be the old-fashioned type, and many women prefer to use the ones they are used to.

   Tampons are never suitable following a hysterectomy or other gynaecological operation, as they increase the risk of infection being introduced into the vagina.

2 *Loose, comfortable underwear.* If your operation has involved a vertical incision, any type of underpants will be uncomfortable for the first few days, and you will probably not wear them. If a catheter has been inserted to drain your bladder of urine, there will be a short length of soft tubing extending from your urethra which can be squashed by tight-fitting pants. Even if you do not have an abdominal wound, high-waisted, loose pants will be more comfortable.

3 *Nightclothes.* Loose, comfortable nightdresses are best. You will be given a hospital shift to wear during the operation itself.

4 *Slippers.*

5 *Dressing gown.*

6 *Towel and washing things.*

7   *Money*. A small amount of money may be useful for newspapers and the telephone. Large sums of money, wallets and handbags should not be taken into hospital as these may have to be kept in an unlocked cabinet by your bed. If you do have to take any valuables or large sums of money into hospital, you should give these to the nurse in charge of your ward when you are admitted. You will be given a receipt listing each item and this should be kept safe so that you can collect your possessions when you are discharged. However, hospital authorities strongly discourage people from bringing anything of great value with them unless absolutely necessary.

8   *Books and magazines*. There will inevitably be periods of waiting between visits from medical staff before your operation, and you may want something to occupy you during this time, as well as during your post-operative stay.

9   *Loose clothing and shoes*. Clothes such as tight jeans will be uncomfortable after your operation, whether or not you have an abdominal wound. Casual, comfortable clothes such as jogging trousers are ideal.

10   *Drugs you are already taking*. Once your admission has been arranged, your GP will have been asked to fill in a form stating all the drugs you are taking and their doses. You may also be asked to take your drugs with you when you go into hospital so that their dosages can be checked and so that you can continue to be given any which are necessary. All your drugs will be kept for you during your stay as you must only take those which are given to you by medical staff. If you are asked to take your own drugs into hospital, these should be returned to you before you leave.

11   *Admission letter*. An admission letter will have been sent to you from the hospital, and you should take this with you when you are admitted for your operation.

Jewellery

Whenever possible, all jewellery should be left at home. Although wedding rings may be worn during an operation, there is a risk that any jewellery you take off before surgery may be lost or stolen. If you have to take any jewellery into hospital, it should be given to the ward sister for safe keeping.

Bleeding during surgery is controlled by **electrocautery**. An electric current is used to heat the tip of an instrument which then shrivels and seals the little blood vessels and stops the bleeding. Therefore wedding rings, or any other rings which are very precious to you or which cannot be removed, will be covered with adhesive tape during surgery as metal can cause electrical burns or electric shocks during this process.

Hospital staff

The ward of a hospital is a busy place and can seem rather confusing and frightening. It may help to have an idea of the different medical staff you are likely to meet, and the jobs they do.

Nurses

The uniforms worn to distinguish nurses of different ranks will vary from hospital to hospital. In some hospitals, the nurses all wear the same uniform, but with their grades indicated by, for example, belts of different colours. All nurses wear badges which state clearly their name and sometimes their grade. There are, of course, both male and female nurses, although women are still in the majority. The nursing grades are as follows.

1   The most senior nurse on the ward is the *ward sister* or *ward manager*. Each ward will have one ward sister who will be very experienced and able to answer any questions you may have. The ward sister has 24-hours a day responsibility for all the staff and patients on at least one ward, for the day-to-day running of the ward, standards of care etc., and is ultimately responsible for the ward even when not on duty. The ward sister will be a registered nurse (RN), who has usually been qualified for at least 5 years. Ward sisters may wear a uniform of a single colour, often dark blue.

　　The male equivalent of the ward sister is a *charge nurse*. Charge nurses often wear a white tunic.

2   When the ward sister is not on duty, there may be a *senior staff nurse* in charge. The senior staff nurse is deputy to, and works closely with, the ward sister. Like the ward sister, this nurse will be very experienced.

3   Each ward may have several *staff nurses*. These are registered nurses who have completed their nursing training. They may be newly qualified or may have several years' experience, and will take charge of the ward when both the ward sister and senior staff nurse are unavailable. There are different grades of staff nurse, each distinguished by a different coloured belt, hat or uniform.

　　The more junior staff nurses are very often in their first or second post since qualifying. They are less involved in ward management, and are therefore able to work closely with the patients. Most of the staff nurses on a ward will be junior staff nurses.

4   *Enrolled nurses* are gradually being replaced. They have undergone 2 years of training and, like the junior staff nurses, are mainly involved in patient care rather than ward management.

5   As student nurses now spend more time in college and less on the wards of hospitals, *health care assistants* (HCAs) have been brought in to take their place. These are unqualified nurses who have undergone 6 months' training on day release while working on a ward and who have then been assessed for a National Vocational Qualification by senior nurses. Health care assistants are able to carry out all basic nursing duties except for the dispensing of drugs. They are supervised at all times by a qualified nurse.

6   The ward may also have several *nursing auxiliaries*. These are not trained nurses, but are present on the ward to deal with any non-medical jobs and to help with the basic care of patients. Their duties include making beds, handing out tea, and putting away linen etc.

7   Student nurses – *diploma nursing students* or *Project* 2000 *students* – are unpaid, and allocated to the wards at various stages during their college-based training. They are mainly involved in observing, and carrying out limited clinical tasks. In their last term before they qualify, they will be rostered on to nursing shifts and be part of a ward team.

Doctors

Each consultant surgeon in a hospital heads a team of doctors of different ranks, sometimes known as a 'firm'. You may meet some or all of them. These doctors can, of course, be men or women.

1   The *consultant surgeon* holds the ultimate responsibility for all the patients on the operating list, and for the work of all the staff in the 'firm'. Consultants have at least 10 to 15 years' experience as surgeons.

You may never actually see the consultant surgeon who is responsible for your care, but you will probably be visited on the ward before your operation by whichever surgeon is to perform it.

2   The *senior registrar* is a very experienced surgeon who has completed several years of training and will soon be appointed to a consultant's post.

3   *Registrars* have trained as surgeons for at least 2 or 3 years and are able to carry out some surgery alone, assisting the consultant, or being assisted by the consultant, on more difficult operations. A registrar is unlikely to perform a hysterectomy alone.

4   Some hospitals employ *clinical assistants* as surgeons. These are often very experienced surgeons who, for personal or family reasons, are not able to work full time. You may not meet this surgeon before your operation.

5   Before your operation you may be examined on the ward by a *senior house officer* (SHO), or by a house surgeon (see below). Senior house officers have been qualified doctors for between 1 and 5 years, and are gaining further experience in hospital before becoming surgeons or specialising in another branch of medicine.

6   A *house surgeon* (or *house officer*) may be directly concerned with your care both before and after your operation, taking notes of your medical history and arranging for any necessary pre-operative investigations to be done, such as a blood count, chest X-ray or electrocardiogram. House officers are qualified doctors who have completed at least 5 years of undergraduate training and are working for a further year in hospital before becoming fully registered doctors. Although house officers do not perform surgery on their own, they may assist the surgeon in the operating theatre.

Anaesthetists are highly trained doctors who specialise in giving anaesthetics and in pain relief. An anaesthetist will also visit you before your operation to discuss any relevant details, such as any anaesthetics you have had in the past and any drugs you may be taking (see Chapter 6).

Medical social workers

If any problems arise at home during your stay in hospital, or if you are concerned about being able to manage on your own once you return home, you can ask to talk to a medical social worker. Medical social workers work in close partnership with other medical staff in the hospital and will be able to give you advice and practical support.

If you or nursing staff feel you will require immediate assistance on leaving hospital, such as 'meals on wheels' or a home help, and you have not been able to discuss this with a social worker during your stay in hospital, the nursing staff can organise this care for you, and can arrange for a social worker to visit you subsequently at home.

Before the operation

Admission to the ward

When you arrive at the hospital, you should report to the main reception desk with your admissions letter. The staff there will check your details and tell you which ward to go to. Once on the ward, the ward clerk will deal with the clerical side of your admission, filling in the necessary forms with you. You will then be allocated a bed and introduced to your **named nurse**.

The **Named Nurse Initiative** was introduced into NHS hospitals under the government's Patients' Charter. A particular nurse is now responsible for planning each patient's nursing care throughout their stay in hospital. (The ward sister will, of course, still be informed of all aspects of your care, and will be able to discuss it with you or your relatives.)

Your 'named nurse' will admit you to the ward, look after you during your stay, and co-ordinate your discharge when the time comes. You will be allocated another nurse for other working shifts. The idea is for people to be identified as individuals who are known to at least one nurse on each shift and who are involved in their own care. To this end, you will be asked to help your nurse draw up a care plan when you are admitted to the ward. You should tell the nurse of any preferences or dislikes you have, for example if you prefer to sleep with several pillows, if there are certain foods you do not want, or if you have any ailments other than that for which you are having surgery, such as arthritis.

Your nurse's name may be displayed above your bed or on your bedside locker so that your relatives and other nursing and medical staff know who to talk to about your care. Your care plan may be kept at the bottom of your bed, but wherever it is, it is available for you to read. Nursing staff may tick off a checklist as they carry out the various procedures and will update the care plan with you as the need arises.

Do tell the nurse if you have any problems or if you are anxious about *any* aspect of your hospital stay.

As you are admitted to the ward, the nurse will take notes of your personal details and explain the ward procedures to you. Your discharge will also be planned at this time. The nursing staff will need to be sure that someone will be able to collect you and take you home when the time comes. If this is not possible, hospital transport can be arranged for you. Before you are due to go home, the nurses will have to be sure you can manage. The effects of anaesthetic gases, and other agents used by the anaesthetist, can stay in your body for several days, and although you may feel you are fully recovered, your reaction times may be slow and you may continue to feel sick and light-headed for at least the next couple of days. Elderly people particularly should have someone to help them for a few days after their operation. All this will be taken into account as you and the nurse plan your discharge.

The nurse will measure your blood pressure, temperature and pulse. A sample of your urine may be taken for analysis to make sure you do not have diabetes or any disorder of the kidneys that would make the operation inadvisable. You will also be weighed as the anaesthetist may need to know your weight in order to be able to calculate the dose of anaesthetic you require.

You will be shown to your bed on the ward and told of any ward details, such as meal times, and where to find the toilets and day room etc.

Anti-embolism stockings

Once you are settled on the ward, a nurse will probably measure your legs for the stockings you will be given to wear during your operation. These **T**hrombo-**E**mbolic **D**eterrent **S**tockings (TEDS) used to be worn only by patients having major operations to help prevent blood clots forming in the veins deep within the legs as they lay motionless on the operating table, sometimes for several hours. However, they are now used routinely as a precaution in almost all operations. Although they may feel uncomfortable, particularly when the weather is hot, there is no doubt as to their value.

The normal activity of the muscles in the legs helps to keep the blood moving through them. During long periods of bed rest or anaesthesia, these muscles are inactive and the circulation of blood in the legs slows down. A blood clot is thus more likely to form which can block the passage of blood through the vein. If pieces of this clot break off, they form **emboli**. Even one embolus may have serious consequences if it travels through the circulation and lodges in a vital organ such as the lung. Anti-embolism stockings improve the return of venous blood to the heart and thus help to prevent blood clots forming.

The nurse will measure your calf and thigh and the length of your leg, and will give you a pair of stockings of the correct size.

If you have a history of varicose veins or thrombosis which increases your risk of developing a blood clot, you will probably have to wear the stockings throughout your hospital stay. Otherwise you will probably not need to put them on until you are preparing to go to the operating theatre. You will be told to keep them on until you are up and about again after your operation.

Heparin injections

At some hospitals, all women undergoing a hysterectomy may be given subcutaneous injections of a low dose of heparin. At others, only high-risk patients, such as those with a previous history of deep vein thrombosis, will have them. Heparin is an anticoagulant, found naturally within the body, which thins the blood and helps to prevent blood clots forming and blocking the blood vessels.

The injections are started with the premedication, and involve the insertion of a very fine needle into the fat – usually on the thigh. They are normally continued, two or three times a day, until you are mobile. Occasionally small bruises can develop around the area of injection.

A worry with this type of surgery used to be that heparin could increase the bleeding, but it does not seem to do so significantly, and heparin injections are very effective in reducing the serious complications of thrombosis and pulmonary embolism.

Antibiotics

It is routine practice in some hospitals to give a dose of antibiotics with the premedication, often via injection into a vein, or via suppositories. These may be continued for 2 to 3 days postoperatively. It is important therefore that you tell the doctor who visits you on the ward before your operation if you are allergic to any antibiotics so that these can be avoided.

Blood samples

Before your operation a blood test will be done to check your level of haemoglobin, and a sample will also be taken to group your blood in case a transfusion is necessary during the operation or afterwards. It is unlikely that you will need a blood transfusion during the operation, but it is possible – this is major surgery.

Visit by the doctor

As has already been mentioned, a house surgeon or senior house officer will visit you on the ward before your operation to take details of your medical history, including any allergies you may have and any drugs you are taking, and to examine you. Your GP may have already filled in a form giving the names and dosages of any drugs you have been prescribed, and you should have been told what to do about these. Do not forget to tell the hospital doctor of any other drugs you have been taking which your GP may not be aware of, such as vitamin supplements, cough medicines, aspirins etc., which are available from the chemist without the need for prescription.

If you normally take a contraceptive pill or hormone replacement tablets, you may have been told to stop these for a time before your operation. If you are still taking them when you enter hospital, for example if you have been called for your operation at short notice, you should tell the doctor. Contraceptive pills used to contain much larger amounts of hormones than do the more modern ones, and these high levels of hormones were sometimes associated with complications from blood clots. The newer pills are almost entirely free from these risks, but some surgeons still prefer their patients to stop taking them for at least a month before surgery.

A medical examination is carried out to identify any illness or infection you may have which could complicate the use of a general anaesthetic. If you are over 50 years of age or a heavy smoker, you will probably have to have a chest X-ray and an electrocardiogram so that any potential anaesthetic complications due to breathing or heart problems can be picked up.

The house surgeon will probably also ask you to sign a consent form if you have not already done so. Although it can be assumed that your consent to the operation is implied by the fact that you have entered hospital willingly, consent forms are widely used. By signing this form you are declaring that your operation has been explained to you and that you understand what it entails and have agreed to it taking place. You are also giving your permission for the doctors to take whatever action they feel to be appropriate should some emergency occur during your operation, and for any necessary anaesthetic to be given to you. Do read this form carefully, and ask the doctor to explain anything you do not understand.

Visit by the surgeon
The surgeon who is to perform your operation is also likely to visit you on the ward to check that all is well.

Visit by the anaesthetist
The anaesthetist will probably come to see you to ask you about anything that may be relevant to the choice of anaesthetic given to you.

Anaesthetics have improved considerably during the last few years, and a 'premed.' is now not always given routinely. If you or your anaesthetist do feel that you are very anxious and need something to relax you, you may be given some form of sedative, by mouth or injection, 1 or 2 hours before the operation. If you enter hospital the day before your operation and think that you will be too anxious to sleep that night, you can, of course, ask the house surgeon or senior house officer for something to help you.

False teeth If you have any false teeth or dental bridges, you should tell the anaesthetist as these will have to be removed before you go into the operating theatre. A broken or loose tooth can be inhaled into the lungs during surgery. You should also point out any of your teeth which are capped or have crowns, although ordinary fillings will not be a cause for concern.

'Nil by mouth'

The term 'nil by mouth' means that neither food nor drink must be swallowed. In order to prevent vomiting and the risk of choking on your vomit while you are anaesthetised, you will be told not to eat or drink anything for about 6 hours before your operation, although you will be able to have a few sips of water with any tablets you need to take. If you are admitted the night before surgery and your operation is the next morning, you will be able to have supper on the ward, but are likely to be told not to eat or drink after midnight. If you enter hospital in the morning and your operation is to be that afternoon, you should not eat or drink for about 6 hours beforehand.

Shaving

Apart from being necessary to give the surgeon a clear view of the area to be operated on, shaving also makes the changing or removal of the adhesive wound covering after the operation a less traumatic experience.

You will probably be given either a disposable razor or clippers to shave your pubic hair. Although hair clippers are preferable, and prevent the skin being 'nicked' by leaving a layer of short hair on it, thus reducing the risk of post-operative infection, they are quite expensive. Disposable razors are therefore more commonly used.

If you are anxious about doing the shaving yourself, do ask a nurse if someone can do it for you. Arthritis of the hands can make this a difficult task. A nurse will probably shave you if you are having a vaginal hysterectomy, as the hair will need to be removed from around the vulva, which is rather tricky to do oneself.

Smoking

If you are a heavy smoker and have not been able to cut down or stop altogether, you will be advised not to smoke in the hours before your operation. It is, of course, much better to stop smoking some months before surgery. The carbon monoxide contained in cigarette smoke poisons the blood by replacing some of the oxygen which is carried in it and which is vital to processes such as wound healing.

Obesity

Obesity also adds to the risk of anaesthesia, and for this reason people who are very overweight should try to lose weight before entering hospital. Indeed, some surgeons will refuse to carry out non-emergency operations on heavy smokers or obese patients as they consider the risks to be too great. However, starting a long, strict diet before your operation may also be inadvisable. The consultant will have assessed your weight when seeing you at your out-patients' appointment, and will probably have given you some guidance at that time.

Waiting

It may seem that you have been admitted to hospital unnecessarily early, and you may find you have to wait on the ward with little to do. Apart from having to be seen by all the medical staff mentioned above, who are responsible for many other patients as well, time will also have been allowed for the assessment of any medical problems you may have, and for the results of any blood tests to be received.

Sometimes operations are cancelled at the last moment. Although this is distressing, and can be very awkward for someone who has had to make special arrangements to come into hospital, it only occurs if an emergency has arisen. Other operations taking place on the same day as yours may be more urgent. If this does occur, you may be sent home and be called again as soon as possible.

You will probably be given only an approximate time for your operation, and be told if it is scheduled for the morning or afternoon. An operation being done before yours may take longer than expected if complications arise.

Leaving the ward

Before being taken from the ward to the anaesthetic room or operating theatre, you will be given a hospital operating gown to wear and will be asked to put on your anti-embolism stockings. A plastic-covered bracelet bearing your name and an identifying hospital number will be attached to one or both of your wrists. You will then be taken from the ward on a hospital trolley.

CHAPTER 6

Anaesthesia

An anaesthetist is a hospital doctor who has been trained in the special skills of giving drugs which cause loss of sensation or consciousness, or both (anaesthetics), and those which block feelings of pain (analgesics). Anaesthesia is a vital part of any operation, and a great deal of time and trouble will be taken to make sure that you receive the anaesthetic which best suits you.

An anaesthetist will visit you on the ward before your operation.

The pre-anaesthetic visit

The main reason for the anaesthetist's visit before your operation is to decide what type of anaesthesia would be safest for you. It also gives you the opportunity to discuss any problems or worries you may have concerning your anaesthesia.

The anaesthetist will ask you questions about any anaesthetics you have had before, any drugs you are taking, and about your general health. It is important that you answer these questions as fully as possible. You should also mention to the anaesthetist if you have any false teeth, as these will have to be removed before your operation to avoid the risk of them being inhaled into your lungs while you are anaesthetised.

If you have had any problems in the past such as an allergy to a particular anaesthetic, it will be helpful if you know the name of the drug concerned or the hospital where the operation was carried out. The appropriate records can then be checked to make sure another type of anaesthetic is used for your operation. You should also tell the anaesthetist if you know of any other member of your family who has reacted against a particular drug, as you may have the same problem.

The anaesthetist may also want to examine you and to look at the results of any tests you have had. There are different types of anaesthetic which can be used (see below), and some health problems will preclude the use of certain ones.

General anaesthetic

This is the most common type of anaesthetic for a hysterectomy or endometrial resection. The drugs used will put you to sleep so that you have no feeling in any part of your body. General anaesthetics can be given in two different ways.

1   An *intravenous anaesthetic* can be injected into a vein via a plastic tube which is inserted into your hand or arm. It will put you to sleep within a few seconds.

2   An *inhalational anaesthetic* is a gas which you breathe in through a face mask. It acts within 1 to 2 minutes. As the use of a face mask can cause some people to panic, it is not normally applied until you are asleep.

During the operation, the anaesthetist will make sure you stay asleep by giving you more drugs as necessary.

Risks of general anaesthesia

People with certain medical conditions, such as heart or lung disease, may not be given general anaesthetics as they are potentially at greater risk.

Some people are afraid of being put to sleep by a general anaesthetic in case they never wake up or suffer brain damage. General anaesthetics are very much safer today than they were even 20 years ago, because of the many advances both in techniques and the drugs used. If you are very concerned about this, do mention it to the anaesthetist, who should be able to reassure you.

Although the risks of general anaesthesia are small, they do have to be borne in mind. (See p. 115 for further discussion.)

Spinal and epidural anaesthetics

These are types of local anaesthetic which can be injected between the vertebrae of the spine, into the space around the nerves in the back. They cause numbness or loss of sensation in the lower part of the body.

The main advantage of epidural and spinal anaesthetics is for people with certain types of medical condition, such as lung or respiratory muscle disease or heart disease, for whom a general anaesthetic carries more risk. Although they are rarely used for abdominal hysterectomies, they are occasionally useful for women having vaginal hysterectomies or endometrial resection.

Other medication

In some hospitals, a premedication drug (premed.) is given routinely to patients to reduce their anxiety before an operation. This is given by mouth, as tablets or a syrup, or by injection several hours before the operation, and will probably make you feel sleepy.

You may be asked whether you would like to have a premed., or you may have to ask for one yourself if you feel anxious and have not been offered one. You can, of course, also say that you do *not* want one if premeds. are given routinely in your hospital. The anaesthetist will be able to discuss this with you.

You may be given any drugs that you normally take, such as diuretics ('water tablets') or drugs to reduce high blood pressure.

The day of the operation

You will be told not to have anything to eat or drink for at least 6 hours before your operation ('nil by mouth'). The reason for this is to prevent the risk of any food or drink left in your stomach when you are anaesthetised causing you to be sick and to choke on your vomit.

While you are still on the ward, you will be given your premed., if you are to have one, and any medicines you normally take. You will then be taken to the operating theatre, probably on a hospital trolley. You may go first into the anaesthetic room or straight into the operating theatre to be given your anaesthetic.

The anaesthetist, or an assistant, will ask you several questions to confirm your identity and make sure that you are the right person in the right place. Your identity bands will also be checked. Many people have many types of operations each day in a hospital, and these checks, which may be repeated, are essential to make sure no mistakes are made.

The anaesthetist will then fit various monitoring devices to watch over you while you are asleep. A probe may be attached to your finger to measure the amount of oxygen in your blood; some sticky pads may be put on your chest so that your heart beat can be recorded on an electrocardiograph; and a cuff may be put around your arm to measure your blood pressure. All these monitoring devices enable the anaesthetist to make sure that the anaesthetic remains effective and that you remain well during surgery.

A plastic cannula will be put into a vein, probably in the back of your hand, and any drugs will be introduced into your body through this.

Once the anaesthetist is happy with the readings from the monitors, your anaesthesia can start.

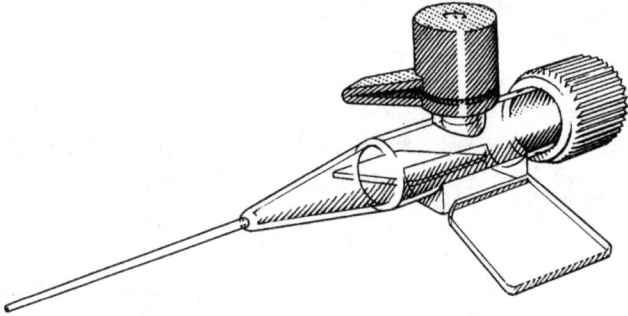

A butterfly cannula. This is a commonly used type of cannula which is inserted into a vein – usually in the back of the hand – and through which drugs can be introduced into the body during an operation.

The anaesthetic

Whatever type of anaesthetic you have, the anaesthetist will remain with you throughout your operation, and may still be there when you wake up.

The anaesthetic will be injected into the tube in your hand or arm, and you will fall asleep within seconds. The drug which makes you go to sleep may sting a little as it enters the vein from the cannula, but this feeling does not last long.

Several different types of drugs will be given to you to make sure you remain asleep and to help you to feel better after your operation:

1 *induction agents* bring on sleep,

2 *maintenance agents* keep you asleep,

3 *analgesics* help to stop you feeling pain after the operation,

4 *anti-emetics* help to stop you feeling sick after the operation.

If local anaesthetic is injected into the wound during your operation to prevent you feeling pain when you wake up, your lower abdomen and groin may be numb for a few hours after surgery.

After your operation

When your operation is over, the anaesthetist will stop giving you the drugs that were keeping you asleep, and you will probably be taken to a recovery room or step-down ward.

The recovery room
The nurses in the recovery room are specially trained to care for patients coming round from anaesthetics after an operation. You will stay in this room, still watched over by monitoring equipment, until you are fully awake and ready to be returned to your own ward.

If you are in pain when you wake up, tell a nurse in the recovery room as you can be given an injection or tablets to relieve this.

Back on the ward
You will be taken back to your own ward, where the anaesthetist will visit you to ensure that you are having adequate pain relief and have no ill-effects from your operation. Do tell the anaesthetist if you have any concerns or questions.

Side-effects of the anaesthetic

There are side-effects which can occur after anaesthesia, but these do not normally last longer than a couple of days. A sore throat is quite common, and is caused by the dry gases breathed while you are asleep, or by the tube which may have been put down your throat to help you breathe during your operation. You may have backache if you have had a spinal or epidural anaesthetic. Both of these side-effects will disappear within a few days.

If you feel unwell, or have pain anywhere other than at the site of your wound, do tell the anaesthetist – or a nurse on your ward – so that the reasons for it can be discovered.

Pain relief

As the effects of any local anaesthetic injected during your operation begin to wear off, you should let a doctor or nurse know as soon as you start to feel pain, so that you can be given some sort of painkiller, either by injection or in the form of tablets.

The amount of pain suffered after a hysterectomy varies from person to person. Some women have pain or slight discomfort for only 12 to 24 hours and will not need any pain-killing injections after this. Others may need injections for up to 3 days after their operation.

Patient-controlled analgesia

One of the newer techniques for relieving post-operative pain is patient-controlled analgesia (PCA). In some hospitals, women may be offered PCA after a hysterectomy. It has proved a good method of pain relief for people with severe pain, although it is not necessary for those whose pain is mild. The PCA machine is expensive, and may not be available for all patients. You can ask a nurse or the anaesthetist at the pre-operative visit if these pumps are available.

As already mentioned, people differ in the amount of pain they feel after similar operations, and different types of operation give rise to different amounts of pain, which can last for varying lengths of time. Thus, one woman may have what she describes as 'mild pain' for only 2 days following a hysterectomy; another may experience 'the worst pain ever' for a week after an identical operation. The technique of PCA has therefore been designed to allow patients themselves to control the amount of pain-relieving drug they receive rather than having to ask a nurse or doctor for an injection or tablets. It generally provides better pain relief than do other more conventional forms of analgesia.

If a PCA machine is available, its workings will be explained to you before your operation. The machine is basically a pump which delivers a pain-killing drug into your body each time you press a button. It is programmed, rather like a computer, to allow you only a safe limit of the drug. The analgesic is usually delivered via a cannula in a vein in your hand or arm, but occasionally may go into the skin of your lower abdomen. Once you press the button, your pain should start to lessen within 5 to 10 minutes. If it does not do so, you should press the button again. As the machine has a built-in safety control to prevent you receiving too much of the drug, you can press the button as often as you like. However, it is important that you do not let anyone else use your machine, as this removes the safety feature.

If, despite pressing the button several times, your pain is not being relieved, you should tell a nurse or doctor on your ward so that the machine can be reset to deliver a stronger dose of the drug – if this is appropriate.

A doctor or nurse will inspect the counter on your machine every day or so to see how many times you have pressed the button and how much of the analgesic drug you have received. Once it is clear that you are reducing the amount of drug you need, and therefore your pain is improving, the machine setting can be changed so that a lower dose is delivered at each press of the button. It will be possible to stop using the machine a day or two later, and to change to another form of pain relief – probably tablets. Patient-controlled analgesia is normally used for 24 to 48 hours after a hysterectomy, and occasionally up to 72 hours.

CHAPTER 7

The operations

Once a decision has been made to go ahead with surgery, the consultant will probably suggest one of four operations: abdominal hysterectomy, vaginal hysterectomy, laparoscopically assisted vaginal hysterectomy, or transcervical resection of the endometrium. Although you may have some say in the choice of procedure, not all operations are technically possible for every woman.

The following are brief descriptions of a typical method used to perform each operation.

Abdominal hysterectomy

When the general anaesthetic has taken effect, you will be transferred to the operating table, lying on your back. A catheter will be passed to empty your bladder of urine, and thus help to avoid it being damaged during the operation. Some surgeons prefer to remove the catheter when the bladder is empty, others leave it in place. The skin around the operating site and your vagina will then be cleaned with an antiseptic solution.

A transverse incision is usually made just below or above the border of the pubic hair, but if your uterus is enlarged or you have had previous abdominal surgery, a vertical cut may be necessary instead.

Once the surgeon has access to your abdominal cavity, your uterus, ovaries and pelvis will be checked for disease.

Before the uterus can be removed, the connective tissue which surrounds it must be divided. Three or four sets of clamps

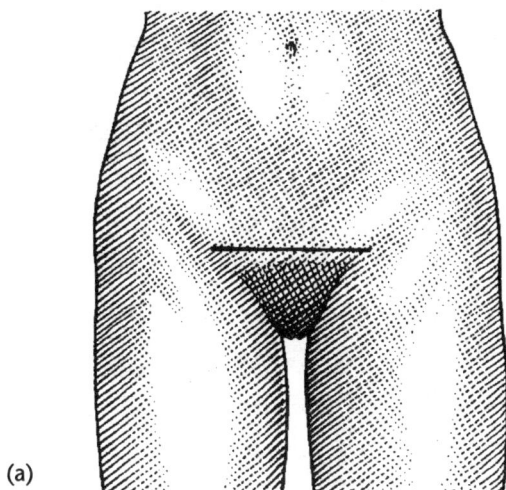

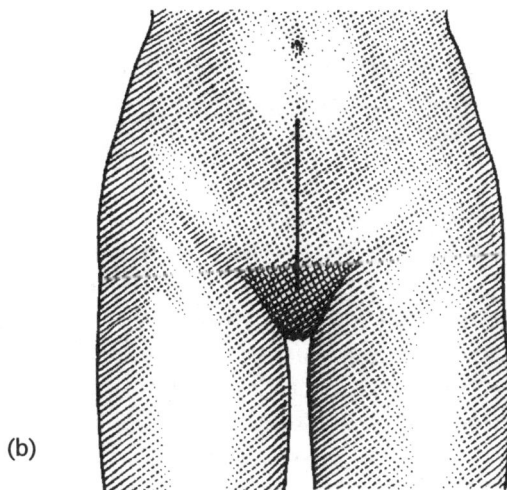

Incisions for an abdominal hysterectomy. (a) A transverse incision is usually used for an abdominal hysterectomy. (b) A vertical incision may be necessary if the uterus is enlarged or there has been previous abdominal surgery.

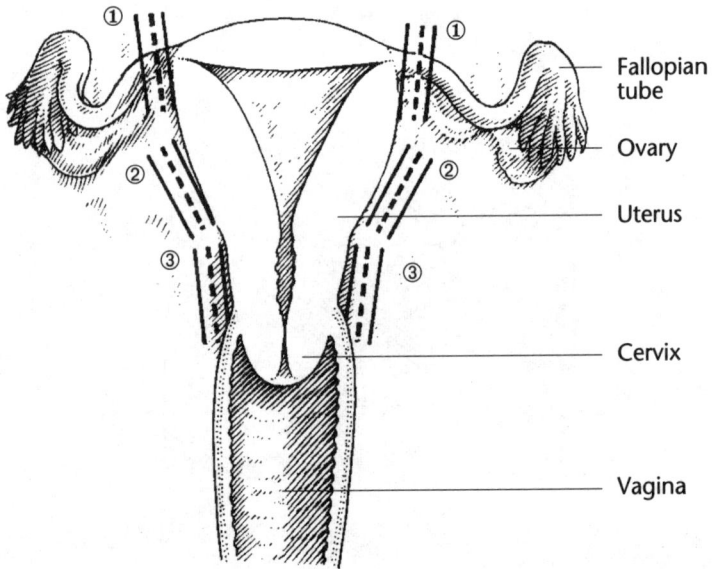

Abdominal hysterectomy. The solid lines represent the positions of clamps placed on either side of the uterus. The broken lines show where a cut is made between each set of clamps to free the uterus from the surrounding connective tissue. The cuts are made in order, from 1 to 3.

are placed in this connective tissue on either side of the body of the uterus and the cervix. The tissue between the topmost pair of clamps on one side of the uterus is cut, and the section of tissue which is to remain (known as a **pedicle**) is tied off securely with absorbable thread to prevent excessive blood loss from it. The process will be repeated on the other side of the uterus, then between the two middle sets of clamps, and finally between the two lowermost sets. Before the second set of clamps is applied, the bladder has to be separated from the uterus and pushed down from its position in front of the body of the uterus and the cervix to allow the vagina to be entered. A cut is made around the circumference of the vagina where it meets the cervix, and the cervix can be pulled out and removed with the rest of the uterus. The top of the vagina is then either over-sewn or its walls are closed with absorbable stitches to prevent further bleeding.

When all bleeding has stopped, the surgeon will close the incision in your abdominal wall. Sometimes as a matter of rou-tine, and sometimes because there is concern about bleeding, suction drains will be left in the pelvis and/or in the abdominal wall to withdraw the blood that collects.

Bilateral salpingo-oophorectomy

This operation to remove the ovaries can often be done at the same time as an abdominal hysterectomy. The clamps are placed in the tissue between the ovaries and the pelvic wall, rather than between the ovaries and the uterus, and the ovaries can then be removed with the uterus.

Sub-total hysterectomy

As the cervix is not removed in this operation, the vagina does not need to be entered. The procedure is similar to that described for abdominal hysterectomy, but less separation of the bladder from the uterus is required as it is not necessary to have access to the cervix in the same way. When the body of the uterus is removed, the cervical stump is left in place, and any remaining endometrium is cored out.

Vaginal hysterectomy

This operation is also similar to an abdominal hysterectomy, but it is performed through the vagina. To release the uterus, the sections of tissue are cut in reverse order, starting with the lowermost pedicle near the vagina. It is not easy to remove the ovaries by this method; they may be felt, but they are not usually visible.

When the general anaesthetic has taken effect, you will be placed on your back on the operating table, with your legs raised up in stirrups – in the **lithotomy position**. Your skin and vagina will be cleaned, and a catheter passed into your bladder. As before, once your bladder is empty, the catheter will either be removed or left in place.

To remove the uterus through the vagina, an incision is made around the cervix. The bladder is separated from the front of the cervix and uterus by a combination of cutting and pushing. A cut is then made through the **peritoneum** (the membrane which lines the abdominal cavity) at the front of the uterus, and in the pocket between the rectum and the back of the uterus, known as the **pouch of Douglas**. The tissue at either side of the uterus is then divided, as described for an abdominal hysterectomy.

If the vaginal walls have prolapsed – either anteriorly as a

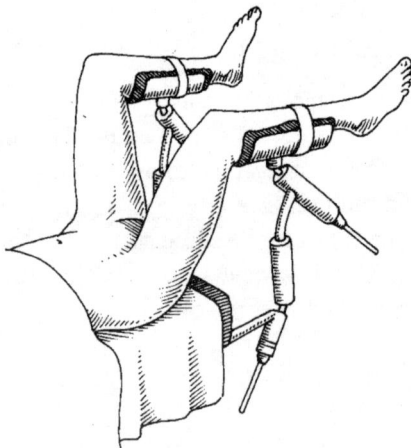

The lithotomy position. To perform a conventional vaginal hysterectomy, or a laparoscopically assisted vaginal hysterectomy, the patient's legs are raised in stirrups, as shown.

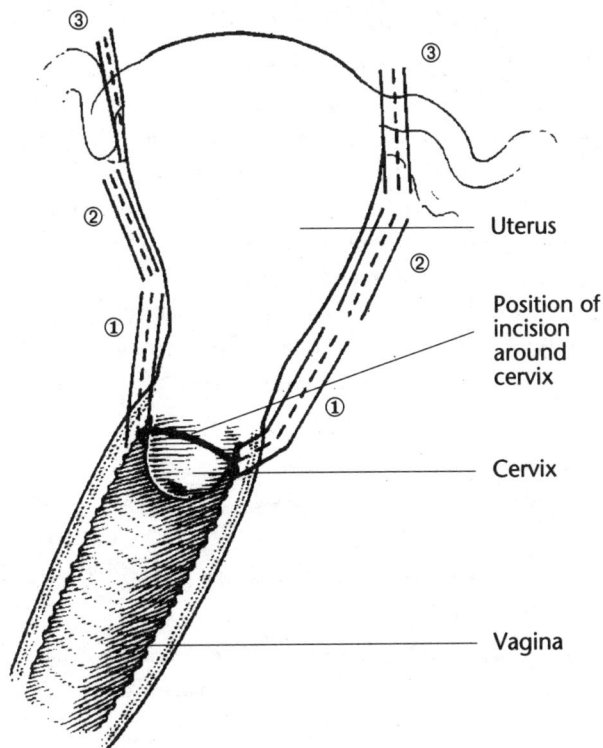

Vaginal hysterectomy. An incision is made around the cervix, as indicated by the solid line. A cut is made between each set of clamps to free the uterus, as for an abdominal hysterectomy but in reverse order, beginning at the bottom of the uterus.

result of the bladder pushing down onto the vagina, or posteriorly due to protrusion of the rectum or bowel – any necessary repair will be made to them before they are closed with absorbable stitches.

Laparoscopically assisted vaginal hysterectomy

A variation of a vaginal hysterectomy may be done using a laparoscope. The recent advances in the design of surgical instruments have enabled a range of operations to be carried out through a series of small incisions rather than through a single larger one. The laparoscope is a type of telescope with a video camera and light source attached. It enables the surgeon to obtain a clear view of the abdominal cavity, a video picture of which is displayed on a screen in the operating theatre. The uterus, fallopian tubes, ovaries and other abdominal structures are thus clearly visible to the surgeon throughout the operation.

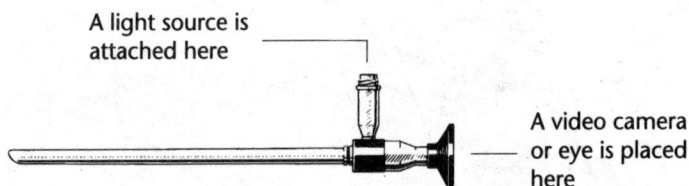

A light source is
attached here

A video camera
or eye is placed
here

A laparoscope. The laparoscope is inserted through a small incision in the abdomen and allows the surgeon to see into the abdominal cavity.

For a laparoscopically assisted vaginal hysterectomy you will be placed on the operating table in the lithotomy position, and a catheter will be passed to empty your bladder.

A small incision will then be made below the umbilicus, and a needle inserted through it. Carbon dioxide gas is pumped through this needle to inflate the abdomen. Electrical instruments are used to stop bleeding during an operation, and these may produce sparks. As carbon dioxide does not support combustion, it will prevent any sparks from igniting. It is not a poisonous gas, and any remaining in the abdomen at the end of the operation will be absorbed by the body and expired by the lungs. A special gas-delivery system is used to keep the abdomen inflated during the operation and thus enable the

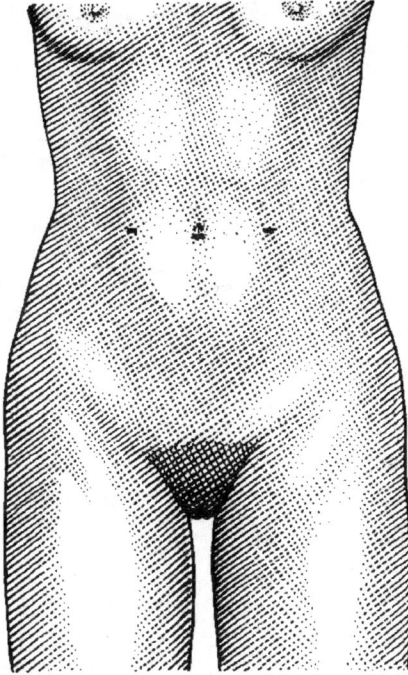

Incisions for laparoscopic hysterectomy. This diagram shows the postions of the three small incisions made in the abdomen and through which the laparoscope and surgical instruments are inserted.

surgeon to have a clear field of vision.

When the abdomen is inflated, a sharp metal instrument called a **trocar** is introduced through the small incision, and the laparoscope is inserted through this. The trocar simply acts as a piloting instrument for the insertion of the laparoscope.

Two more trocars are then inserted to the right and left of the uterus through which instruments can be passed. Rather than having to insert clamps and then cut between them, as in an open operation, the surgeon will use a **linear stapler** which automatically staples and cuts the upper two pedicles. The metal staples effectively secure the cut surface of the tissue and prevent further bleeding.

The surgeon then washes out the abdominal cavity with a saline solution passed through a trocar. The saline and any blood are withdrawn in the same manner. Other instruments will also be pushed through the trocars to dissect the bladder away from the uterus, as in conventional open surgery.

The operation is completed by cutting the skin at the top of the vagina, as in a vaginal hysterectomy, dividing one pedicle at either side of the cervix, and pulling the uterus gently out through the vagina.

The incisions which are made for laparoscopic surgery are very small, and the recovery time is shorter than that following conventional surgery. However, the operation itself does take longer than a similar open operation, and therefore the period of anaesthesia is longer.

Transcervical resection of the endometrium (TCRE)

The endometrium can either be destroyed by **endometrial ablation**, which involves the use of a laser or electrocautery to burn it away, or it can be cut out in strips by **endometrial resection**. There is no proven advantage to using the laser technique, and the operation may take longer if done this way. As ablation or resection of the endometrium is a more minor procedure than a hysterectomy, it can often be done as a day case.

Transcervical resection of the endometrium is only possible if your uterus is not enlarged and if your cervix can be dilated to insert the **resectoscope** (see below). The endometrium must have been prepared before the operation, as described on p. 38.

Once the general anaesthetic has taken effect, you will be placed on the operating table in the lithotomy position and your vagina will be cleaned. Your cervix will then be dilated to allow the resectoscope to be inserted without causing any damage.

The resectoscope consists of a ridged metal tube containing fibre-optic fibres connected to a lens system and powerful light source. Around it are inflow and outflow sheaths that allow fluid to be pushed into the uterine cavity where it circulates before being sucked out. The fluid is used to distend the uterine cavity, thus allowing the surgeon a clear field of vision. The lenses connected to the resectoscope remain outside the body, where they are linked to a viewing camera.

Once the resectoscope is in the uterine cavity, the surgeon will look for signs of disease such as polyps, fibroids and cancer. If all appears to be normal, the process of ablation or resection of the endometrium can begin, aiming to remove the entire endometrium and one-third of the myometrium. At the end of the procedure the surgeon will check that no accessible endometrium has been missed and that there is no excessive bleeding.

During the operation a strict check is kept on the amount of fluid entering and leaving the uterine cavity. If more than 1 litre of fluid is unaccounted for, the operation will be stopped to avoid the risk of the **intoxication syndrome** developing. This can occur if excess water and sodium are absorbed by the body, and can lead to mental confusion and heart failure.

CHAPTER 8

After your operation: in hospital

This chapter gives details of what is likely to happen from the time you leave the operating theatre until you are discharged from hospital.

Blood transfusion

If heavy bleeding occurred during your operation, a blood transfusion may be necessary. Bleeding during surgery is known as **primary bleeding,** and surgeons have to deal with it in whatever way seems appropriate. Blood transfusions are only given during an operation if essential, but if you have strong views about them, you should make these known to the surgeon beforehand. After the operation, when you are conscious, the surgeon will discuss with you whether you need a blood transfusion or simply iron replacement tablets or injections.

The recovery room

Once your operation is over, you will be taken to the recovery room, where you will remain until you are fully awake. A trained nurse will be present while you are unconscious to keep a close check on your recovery from the anaesthetic. When the nurses are satisfied that your operation seems to have been successful and that there is no excessive bleeding or other complications, a nurse will come to collect you, and a hospital porter will wheel you back to your ward on a trolley or mobile bed. If the nurses on the ward are busy and do not feel that they will be able to provide satisfactory care, your return to the ward may be delayed.

After an abdominal hysterectomy, in particular, you may feel some pain, and the recovery nurse will probably give you pain-killing injections as you need them. Do ask for these if you are in pain and they have not been offered to you.

Drips and drains

When you come round from the anaesthetic, you may have the following devices attached to you.

Intravenous drip

After any form of hysterectomy you will have an intravenous drip, usually going into your wrist but possibly higher in your arm. This is to replace the fluids that were lost from your body during the operation. You may feel thirsty when you come round from the anaesthetic but, to avoid the risk of vomiting, will not be able to have anything to drink, although you may be given a mouthwash. The fluid you need is going into your body through the drip. Blood can also be given by this route if necessary.

Urinary catheter

If you have had a hysterectomy, a catheter may have been inserted through the urethra into your bladder. A catheter is a small, flexible tube which is coated with local anaesthetic before being passed through the urethra. Although this may sound a painful process, it is less so than having a blood test.

If the catheter has been left in place at the end of your operation, it will probably be attached to your leg to avoid any jerking movements pulling on it and hurting your sensitive urethra. Once a catheter has been inserted into the bladder, it is held in place by a balloon which is inflated with a small amount of fluid.

Before the catheter is removed, a nurse will let this fluid out so that the balloon goes back to its original size.

A full bladder is uncomfortable, and therefore some surgeons leave the catheter in place routinely; others only when they think it is necessary.

Very rarely, the bladder is damaged during an operation and a catheter is then essential to allow it to heal.

Draining excess blood

Drains may be put into the pelvis or into the wound. There are various types available which usually consist of a thin plastic tube attached to a plastic bottle with suction. These drain any excess blood which may collect after the operation, and which, if it was left in the body, could lead to an infection and fever.

The drains also allow the surgeon to monitor the amount of internal bleeding occurring post-operatively. Small amounts of bleeding are inevitable and are dealt with effectively by the body.

Following your operation you may therefore have one or two drains – or possibly none at all – depending on how the operation has gone and on your surgeon's routine practice.

Vaginal packs

There is always some vaginal bleeding following all the different operations. If this is heavier than a period, it may be significant. A pad may have been placed between your legs when you were unconscious, and the nurses will check this from time to time until you are fully awake and able to do it for yourself.

During a vaginal hysterectomy, a pack may be inserted into the vagina to absorb the blood. The pack is soaked in an anti-septic cream, usually yellow or white in colour, and it will probably be removed the next day (see below). If bleeding from the vagina is heavy, the pack may be left in place a little longer. It is only after the pack has been removed that bleeding is likely to be obvious.

If you do have a vaginal pack, you will probably also have a catheter as the pack will put pressure on the adjacent urethra, and may cause slight discomfort.

After a hysterectomy

When you return from the recovery room, you will be lifted into your bed and, if you are wearing any rings, the tape will be removed from them. You may remain in the operating gown until the following day.

The anaesthetic will probably have made you feel light headed and very sleepy. You may feel nauseated and, because a tube has been passed down your throat during anaesthesia, you may have a dry or sore throat. To avoid the risk of vomiting, you will not usually be given anything to eat or drink until the day after an abdominal hysterectomy, but you can request a mouthwash. Following a laparoscopic or vaginal hysterectomy, you may be able to have a few sips of water, but this will depend on the surgeon's instructions to the nurses.

During the first 2 hours after your operation your blood pressure and pulse will be checked frequently.

If you suffer any discomfort, do tell a nurse.

The first post-operative day is the most painful and difficult one. You will be very tired and want to sleep a lot. Your visitors should be limited to members of your immediate family, who should not stay too long.

Removal of the vaginal pack

If you have a vaginal pack, and your blood loss is not heavy, this will be removed by a nurse in the first 24 hours after surgery. As your vagina may be dry, and the removal of the pack is an uncomfortable procedure, you will first be given an intramuscu-

79

lar pain-killing injection. Once the pack has been removed, you will have to remain in bed for a couple of hours, during which time any blood loss will be checked for at regular intervals.

Explanations and questions

During the first post-operative day, the surgical team may visit you on the ward and the surgeon will explain to you exactly what happened during the operation. You will also be examined. The surgeon will have seen you after the operation and, if you were awake, will have spoken to you. However, it is very common for people not to remember what is said to them just after an anaesthetic, so the surgeon will probably repeat everything the following day. There will be other opportunities to ask questions, but this is a good time to ask any about the operation itself. Questions about subsequent hormone replacement therapy etc. can wait until you feel a little stronger, but do ask at this time if you wish.

Painkillers

During the first few post-operative hours, you will probably have been given a strong painkiller such as morphine, which causes the unfortunate side-effects of nausea, headache and vomiting. This will have been adminsitered by intramuscular injections, by a continuous intravenous pump, or possibly by a patient-controlled pump (see p. 64). If you have a continuous intravenous pump, you should tell a nurse or doctor if you feel nauseated so that the dose being administered can be reduced. Analgesics supplied by a pump system can be continued for 36 to 48 hours.

From day 1 onwards, any analgesic injections will gradually be stopped and tablets or syrup substituted. Suppositories are particularly useful following pelvic surgery as their analgesic effect lasts for a long time and their absorption is good, usually better than oral absorption immediately after an abdominal operation.

If you have had an epidural or spinal anaesthetic, its effect may begin to wear off and your pain may increase. Alternative forms of pain relief should now be substituted.

During the ward visit, the surgeon will check that you are receiving adequate pain relief.

The bowels

The surgeon will ask you if you are feeling sick, and will examine your abdomen and use a stethoscope to listen for the tinkling sounds which can be heard if the bowels are working properly. The bowels often stop working and become slightly distended with fluid and gas after abdominal surgery, but they should start to function normally again after a few days, particularly once you are eating your regular diet and are more active. You may need to take a laxative for a few days after your operation. Your bowels are unlikely to be affected following a laparoscopic hysterectomy, which is one of the reasons recovery is quicker following this type of operation.

After laparoscopic hysterectomy, you will probably be allowed to eat and drink normally. If you have passed urine and the surgeon is satisfied with your general state, you may be allowed to go home during the day after your operation. This is not normally possible following an abdominal or vaginal hysterectomy.

Eating and drinking

Once your bowels are working – which may only take a few hours – you will be able to start taking sips of water, gradually increasing the amount, and then having tea or coffee. Some people prefer to drink tea rather than water, and the nurses will probably agree to this. The important thing is to increase your intake of fluids slowly. If you rush it, you will inevitably feel sick and this can delay your ultimate recovery.

After an abdominal or vaginal hysterectomy, you should not expect to eat anything more than a clear soup on the first post-operative day. On the second day you will probably be able to eat a sloppy diet, and on the third you can eat normally. You are unlikely to feel particularly hungry for the first few days: eat as and when you feel like it. Do not worry if you feel sick – it will be because your bowels and stomach are not quite ready.

Although nutrition is important in recovery, it is your nutrition over years, not just a few days, which matters. You will recover just as quickly if you eat nothing during the first few days as you will if you manage a normal diet.

During your check-up on the first post-operative day, the surgeon will give instructions to nursing staff about the fluid to be put into your drip. The drip will probably be taken down once you are drinking normally and not feeling sick.

Passing urine

If your operation has gone well and there has not been any damage to the bladder or excessive bleeding, the urinary catheter, if it has been left in place, will normally be removed on the first post-operative day so that you can try to pass urine, which you will almost certainly be able to do. If not, the catheter will be put back in.

If you do not have a catheter, and have not passed urine during the first post-operative night, the surgeon will try to feel your bladder by pressing on your abdomen, although this is difficult. If you have still not passed urine by mid-morning, a catheter will probably be inserted. Approximately 10% of women are unable to pass urine spontaneously after a hysterectomy.

Bleeding

The surgeon will check that you are not bleeding from the wound site, into the drains or vaginally. You will probably be asked when your sanitary towel was last changed, and the surgeon may want to inspect this to make sure you are not bleeding too heavily.

If heavy bleeding occurs during the first post-operative night, you may be returned to the operating theatre for it to be stopped. Excessive bleeding during the first 36 hours after surgery is most likely to require surgical intervention. After this time, return to theatre will probably not be necessary, and any minor bleeding will gradually lessen.

Depending on the amount of blood in your drains, they may be taken out on the first, second or third post-operative day.

Following an abdominal or vaginal hysterectomy, you will feel much better by the second day, and by the third you should be able to walk up and down the ward several times. You should also be able to start the pelvic floor exercises which the physio-therapist will discuss with you (see p. 104).

You will probably be able to go home between days 3 and 7 after an abdominal or vaginal hysterectomy. Each day you will be visited by a doctor – probably a registrar or house officer – and you may see the full surgical team on at least one other occasion before your discharge from hospital. Do ask to speak to the consultant if you have any particular difficulties to discuss.

Each day the doctors and nurses will make sure that you are eating and drinking appropriately, that you are passing urine and that you are not bleeding excessively. They will want to know that you are moving about and will ask about your bowel motions.

With a vaginal hysterectomy, you may also have had an ante-rior or posterior repair. Posterior repairs, particularly, tend to be more painful and make it more difficult to pass urine. Anterior repairs may also make passing urine difficult as the surgeon has actually been pushing on the bladder.

Emotional ups and downs

Many women find that they weep easily in the first few days after a hysterectomy. The nurses are likely to be sympathetic about this, and you should soon start to feel more cheerful. It is gener-ally recognised that some women feel saddened by what may be an abrupt end to their child-bearing years, and many go through a grieving period similar to that following a loss or bereavement. It is also possible that the changes in the body's hormones following the removal of the womb may play a part in this.

You and your family should be prepared for this possibility, and should try to remember that it is a normal reaction that will probably soon pass.

Vaginal bleeding

Vaginal bleeding will continue if you have had an abdominal or vaginal hysterectomy, and you should have brought a supply of sanitary pads into hospital with you. You will be advised not to use tampons to avoid encouraging any infection. Many hospitals supply rather old-fashioned sanitary pads, and women often feel more comfortable with their own brand.

The bowels

When your bowels do start to work, you will pass wind. It is important that you do not try to hold this in, as letting it out will help speed your recovery. It is a good, positive sign, so do not be embarrassed when asked about it by the doctor. Many women are surprised to find that wind is the main cause of their discomfort after an abdominal hysterectomy – more so than their abdominal wound. Regular painkillers should help.

When your bowels are working properly again, you will have a bowel motion. If you have not done so by day 3, you may be offered a suppository and, as the earlier your bowels are open, the better you will feel, it is probably a good idea to accept it. If you have still not had a bowel motion by day 4 or 5, you may be prescribed some mild purgatives.

The wound

If you have had an abdominal hysterectomy, your abdominal wound will be covered with an adhesive, probably transparent, dressing. The wound may have been closed with several little stitches or one long one under the skin. The stitches may be absorbable, but if not they may be removed, probably about 6 to

7 days post-operatively, by a nurse on the ward, or you will be told to make an appointment for this to be done by the practice nurse at your doctor's surgery.

Before you are discharged, a doctor will inspect your wound to make sure that there is no infection.

By the third day after your operation, your wound dressing can probably be removed and, if the wound looks healthy, you may be able to have a bath. You are unlikely to need to have another wound dressing after this time, but should make sure you keep the wound as dry and clean as possible.

Mobilisation

During and after your stay in hospital, mobilisation is important as it helps to reduce the risk of thrombosis (see p. 110). You should make an effort as soon as possible to walk up and down the ward. If you leave the ward, do tell a senior member of the nursing staff that you intend to do so.

You will probably be able to get out of bed and walk a little on the second post-operative day. After the third day, you should be reasonably mobile.

Compression stockings

Compression stockings are routinely used in many hospitals (see p. 51); in others they are only given to people who are at particular risk of developing deep vein thrombosis (i.e. obese or elderly patients) or those with a previous history of this condition. You may be able to remove your stockings by day 3 after your operation, or may be told to keep them on until you are discharged from hospital.

Heparin injections

If you have been having heparin injections (see p. 52), these will probably be continued until you are mobile.

Antibiotics

If you have been given antibiotics, as is routine practice in some hospitals, these may be continued for 2 or 3 days after your operation.

Blood samples

Post-operatively, usually on day 2, a blood sample will be taken to check how much blood you may have lost. The surgeon will probably know if your haemoglobin level has dropped significantly, and will have asked you about any symptoms of anaemia, such as headache, palpitations or feeling faint.

If you have a haemoglobin level of around 8 g/dl or below (the normal range is 11–15 g/dl), you may be asked if you would like a blood transfusion before you leave hospital or if you would prefer to take iron tablets. Iron tablets need to be started as soon as your bowels are moving, and will have to be continued for 1 to 2 months. If you do have these instead of a transfusion, your haemoglobin level will slowly build up. It *is* a slow process and you will feel very tired and possibly have more difficulty concentrating for a week or so, but apart from minor bowel complications, there are no serious side-effects associated with taking iron tablets.

Blood transfusion will make you feel better within a few hours and will speed your recovery. All blood given in the UK is tested, e.g. for HIV and hepatitis. However, some people develop an allergic reaction to the transfused blood, and you may prefer not to take up this option.

Pain relief

By the time you go home, you will probably be taking oral painkillers once or twice a day and, if you wish, a supply may be given to you. The tablets prescribed in hospital are slightly stronger than paracetamol but may be supplemented with paracetamol if required. You may need oral painkillers for the next few days, at least before you go to bed at night to give you a pain-free night's sleep.

Pain is greater following an abdominal hysterectomy, but

vaginal hysterectomy is also a major operation and, although you will have no external scars to show it has taken place, you will still feel very tired and have some degree of pain.

Hormone replacement therapy (see also p. 8)

If you are pre-menopausal and your ovaries have been removed at the same time as your hysterectomy, the surgeon will probably discuss hormone replacement therapy with you. Hormone replacement is necessary to prevent you becoming abruptly menopausal. The surgeon may have put an implant into your wound at the time of the operation, and you will then need to decide whether you wish to have another implant in 3 months time or start taking tablets or using patches. You therefore have time to consider your treatment options before starting this therapy. If no implant has been inserted before you leave hospital, you will need to start oral medication or patches. It is important that these are continued until at least the time when you would have gone through your menopause naturally. A continuous supply can be obtained through your GP.

After endometrial resection

When you come round after this operation you may or may not have a drip. Drains and catheters are unlikely to have been required, and post-operative retention of urine is unusual. You may have a little difficulty passing urine, and possibly have a burning sensation when you do if a catheter was passed into your bladder.

You will be returned to the ward quite soon – to a day ward if you are going home the same day. You will be able to have something to drink as soon as you want it, starting with a few sips and gradually building up your fluid intake. You will probably be offered a light meal before you go home.

As no cut has been made, you will only need pain-killing tablets or syrup, and are unlikely to have had any injections of morphine. Mild crampy pains are the worst that you are likely to suffer.

There are no stitches following an endometrial resection, but you will inevitably have some bleeding and discharge, and will only be allowed home if these are light. Vaginal bleeding and discharge may stop within a day or two. Sometimes the bleeding following this operation is like a light period; sometimes it can continue, becoming less heavy, until after a week or two it is merely spotting. The spotting may persist for a month, or, in some rare cases, up to 3 months. You should wear sanitary pads rather than tampons while you have a discharge to avoid infection.

You will not have needed compression stockings or be given heparin as you are not immobilised by this operation.

If you do go home on the day of your operation, someone should stay with you during the night in case you have a haemorrhage – which is unlikely but possible.

Discharge letter

Before you leave hospital, you will be given a discharge letter to take to your GP's surgery as soon as possible. The letter will provide your GP with details of your treatment and of whether or not you have stitches that will need to be removed.

Driving

It is not safe to drive home after any of these operations, and you should make arrangements for someone to collect you from hospital when you are discharged.

CHAPTER 9

After your operation: at home

The convalescent beds in nursing homes which were once used for people recovering from major surgery are no longer available under the NHS. There are still convalescent homes for those who are able to pay for their stay. Elderly women would perhaps benefit from a couple of weeks' convalescence as recovery is likely to be slower in this age group. However, for most women, a sensible approach to how much they do, and a gradual increase in their activity should see them through their recovery period.

The arrangements for your care once you leave hospital will have been discussed with you on admission. The nursing staff may be able to tell you if any assistance is likely to be available to you, such as 'meals on wheels' and a home help for elderly women living alone or with an elderly relative. If necessary, you will probably have a chance to talk to a medical social worker about this before you are discharged from hospital. If you are to receive help of this kind, nursing staff may contact the social services a couple of days before you are discharged so that preparations can be made for your care. If the doctors or nurses do not think you are ready to go home at the appointed time, arrangements may be made for you to stay in hospital for an extra day or so.

When you leave hospital you should take with you your discharge letter, any drugs you have been given, such as antibiotics and painkillers, and any valuables or drugs which have been kept for you.

After a hysterectomy

Vaginal bleeding and discharge

Vaginal bleeding will gradually decrease during the following month or so. If it continues for longer, you should consult your doctor.

You may also notice some discharge which is probably coming from the wound at the top of the vagina as it heals. Occasionally there is a profuse discharge from areas of healing tissue, and your doctor may cauterise these by dabbing them with a silver nitrate stick. This is not a painful procedure. Infection may also cause a profuse discharge, and this will need treatment with antibiotics.

During the first few weeks at home, some women bleed fairly heavily and continually and then have a big discharge of blood, after which bleeding stops. Others may bleed very little and then have a sudden large discharge. However, most women have heavy bleeding initially which gradually tails off. A sudden heavy bleed is likely to be due to the escape of blood which has been trapped at the top of the vagina – in a **vault haematoma** (see p. 108). Once the haematoma has discharged you are likely to feel much better. Dark red or brown blood is old blood and it is much better that it comes out. If bleeding does not stop, and particularly if the blood is bright red, and therefore fresh, you should seek advice from your doctor immediately. This type of bleeding may be related to persistent infection.

Stitches

If you have had an abdominal hysterectomy and your stitches are not absorbable, they will probably be taken out before you leave hospital. Otherwise, the nurse at your doctor's surgery will remove them by about 7 to 10 days after your operation, and you will have to make an appointment to have this done.

With a vaginal hysterectomy, you will have had many stitches inside which are all absorbable.

The wound

Following an abdominal hysterectomy, the abdominal wound may be red and noticeable at first, and you may be able to feel some tender lumps under it where it is healing. Unless you have had any complications (see Chapter 11), your wound will be becoming less prominent by about 6 weeks, and by 12 weeks after your operation it will have healed fully and only be a fine pink line, which may be hidden where the pubic hair is growing back. By 6 months, the scar will have become a fine white line.

Bladder and bowel function

If you are taking iron, you may either be constipated or have diarrhoea. For a while after any type of hysterectomy, you may have a burning sensation when you pass urine, but this will probably have resolved before you leave hospital. If you do have difficulty passing urine, or with your bowel motions, you should discuss this with your doctor.

Diet

It is important to have a good healthy diet and to avoid putting on too much weight by eating more than necessary while you are less active. A diet high in fibre will help your bowels to get back to normal.

Exercise

After an abdominal hysterectomy, and to a lesser extent after a vaginal hysterectomy, when you leave hospital you will be fully recovered from the anaesthetic, but as you have had major surgery you may feel weak and tired and unable to do as much as normal. Although you should not stay in bed for long periods of time, it may be better to get up later in the mornings, take a nap in the afternoons, and go to bed earlier at night.

From the first day after your operation you can take mild exercise, gradually increasing the amount of walking you do. Daily short walks are advisable, and you can go shopping when you think you can manage it. But do take someone with you to lift and carry heavy shopping bags.

Driving
It is better to avoid driving a car until you feel it is safe to do so, probably not for at least 2 to 3 weeks, by which time short, local drives should be possible. Long journeys should not be attempted while you still get tired easily. When you do start driving again, you should be able to do an emergency stop if necessary, and can practise this in a stationary car. Use your own judgement to assess when *you* feel confident that you can stop in an emergency, and that you can concentrate sufficiently not to be a danger to yourself or to other road users.

Housework
For the first week after your operation, you will find it a great help to have someone to make meals and do the housework. You will probably be able to make light meals and cups of tea, but will not feel like standing cooking for long periods of time. Many women are concerned because they have heard that they should do *nothing* until at least their 6-week post-operative check-up. This is not the case. Just follow your own instincts and gradually build up what you do as you feel able.

You can gradually increase the amount of housework you do as you start to feel better. The important thing is to avoid lifting *heavy* weights – carrying the vacuum cleaner upstairs, moving furniture etc. – but it is quite all right to lift a kettle. Toddlers can be heavy, and each mother has to decide for herself what she wants to do about lifting them.

During weeks 2 to 6 you will gradually be returning to doing housework, driving, less strenuous sports, and looking after your children.

Returning to work

From 6 to 12 weeks you may still be off work, particularly if your job is a physical one, although some women feel fit to return before this time. But by 3 months, unless there have been complications, you should be fully recovered. There is no medical reason why you should not return to work as soon as you feel fit to do so. If in doubt, discuss this with your GP.

Sexual intercourse

Sexual intercourse can be resumed from any time after 6 weeks, but should be gentle to begin with. If you want to have sexual intercourse before this, you should do so with care. Many women find that sex is never quite the same after a hysterectomy, but most get used to this after a while, and it does not normally lessen their enjoyment.

After laparoscopically assisted hysterectomy

Vaginal bleeding and discharge

Bleeding after laparoscopic hysterectomy is similar to that following other forms of hysterectomy (see above).

Stitches

The stitches in your small abdominal wounds will be absorbable and will gradually dissolve. You may have been told to make an appointment for the practice nurse at your GP's surgery to check these.

Getting back to normal

Because laparoscopic hysterectomy does not involve a large incision, you can expect to get back to normal after 2 to 3 weeks, and return to work some time after this.

You will feel tired after the anaesthetic, perhaps as if you were recovering from flu, and you will have mild abdominal discomfort. You should gradually increase your activity over a couple of weeks as you feel able to do so.

The advice concerning sexual intercourse is the same as that following a vaginal or abdominal hysterectomy (see p. 93).

After endometrial resection

It will probably take you 2 or 3 days to get over the anaesthetic, and you can expect to resume your normal activities and think about returning to work within 1 to 2 weeks after your operation. It is important that you move about as soon as possible to avoid the risk of thrombosis in the leg veins.

There should be no reason not to be mobile once you have got over the effects of the anaesthetic, and you can resume driving at this time. As there are no cuts or wounds, there is no problem with lifting children or doing housework.

Your periods may stop completely after an endometrial ablation or resection, or you may continue to bleed much more lightly at the time of your period. If you have had painful periods due to the passage of clots, the pain is likely to have resolved completely. If the pain was due to endometriosis, it may continue at the time you would have had your period.

Following endometrial resection, there is always the risk of recurrence of your menstrual problems. If your periods continue to be unsatisfactory, you can consider taking medication, having another endometrial resection, or having a hysterectomy. About 1 in 10 women will require further treatment during their lifetime.

The post-operative check-up

After a hysterectomy
Some consultants like all their patients to be seen either by themselves or a member of their team within 6 weeks of a hys-

terectomy. Others prefer GPs to do this follow-up examination. If you do have any problems before your check-up, you can contact the hospital out-patients' department or your consultant's secretary, and an appointment can be made for you if necessary.

At the check-up, apart from having a physical examination, you will be given advice about resuming sexual intercourse, if you have not already done so, and about returning to work and driving.

Making your appointment If your GP is a man, you should explain to his receptionist when you make your appointment that it is for a check-up following a hysterectomy. This is important so that a female surgery nurse can be present during any gynaecological examination, as most male doctors will not do this alone.

After endometrial resection
Following an endometrial resection, your check-up will not be until about 4 months after your operation to allow a true assessment to be made if you have had periods post-operatively.

Holidays

Women often ask if and when they can go on holiday after having had a hysterectomy. A holiday is a good idea, but it is probably better not to leave the country until at least 6 weeks after major surgery of this sort. It is also advisable not to travel to any country which does not provide first-rate medical care for at least 3 months after your operation. After 3 months, if there have been no complications, there is no reason why you should not travel abroad.

Depression

Some women feel depressed for a while after a hysterectomy, but this is less likely to be a problem for those who have been able to make their own decision to have this operation.

It is not uncommon for women to go through an emotional period following a hysterectomy when they are prone to crying and feeling sad. This usually passes within a few days, particularly once they begin to feel the benefits of no longer having painful or heavy periods. It is a natural reaction to the operation, perhaps because it is seen as a sign of getting older, or as a sudden end to your reproductive life if you have not reached your menopause. To decide not to have any more children is one thing, but to know that you cannot is perhaps another. This is something that women face at the menopause, but many women who have a hysterectomy before this time may have to deal with it earlier. You will feel weak and tired for several days after the operation, and this may also contribute to your feelings of depression.

Some women feel less than a complete woman following a hysterectomy. However, the uterus is mainly a container for a developing fetus; your 'womanliness' is built into every part of your body. If the ovaries have not been removed, they will still produce the female hormones in the same cyclical fashion after hysterectomy.

Psychological problems can arise if a hysterectomy is done at a time when a marriage or partnership is rocky, for example when things are wrong with the relationship and the couple's sex life is not good because the woman is bleeding all the time. If the woman has a hysterectomy to improve their sex life, but other factors in the marriage deteriorate, her partner may blame her for being 'no good as a woman', or she may blame herself. Things therefore get worse and worse.

If you have a hysterectomy when you are having an active and regular sex life, you will need the support of your partner, and it is not ideal to have this operation if your relationship is rocky. Your doctor may be able to arrange for you to discuss any problems of this sort with a counsellor if you wish to do so.

A hysterectomy is a major operation and an emotional one. It is particularly important not to undergo any of these procedures if you have any doubts about having completed your family.

Support groups

After a hysterectomy, some women feel that they are 'no longer women' and fear that they are less attractive to their partners. These are common worries, and it does help to discuss them. If depression continues, and you would like support and the chance to talk through your problems with someone who understands, there are support groups which can help you. If there is no local support group in your area, your GP should be able to arrange for you – and your partner if he wishes to – to talk to a counsellor.

Support groups have been set up around the country, mostly by women who have had a hysterectomy themselves. These are normally able to provide information – before and after your operation – and emotional support, by phone, in group meetings or by putting you in contact with someone in your area.

Details of hysterectomy support groups can be obtained from:

Women's Health & Reproductive Rights Information Centre (WHRRIC)
52 Featherstone Street
London EC1Y 8RT
Telephone: 071 251 6580

CHAPTER 10

Some post-operative exercises and tips

While you are in hospital, you may be given notes on how to do some exercises that will help to strengthen your muscles after your hysterectomy, with explanations of why these are important. If you have any breathing problems, you are likely to be visited on the ward by a physiotherapist who will examine your chest and advise you about breathing exercises. You may also have the opportunity while you are still in hospital to attend a session run by a physiotherapist who will explain all the exercises you need to do, and why.

This chapter gives brief details of the most important post-operative exercises, and describes ways of carrying out some normal, everyday activities which you may find difficult in the first few days or weeks after your hysterectomy.

Breathing exercises

You should start doing breathing exercises on the first post-operative day.

During any period of inactivity, such as after an operation when you are in bed or sitting in a chair for most of the day, your breathing will be shallow. Taking deep breaths in and out – at least five times an hour while you are awake – will help air to reach all parts of your lungs and keep them fully expanded.

You should continue the breathing exercises until you are up and walking around the ward. They may also help to lessen any feeling of nausea.

Improving your blood circulation

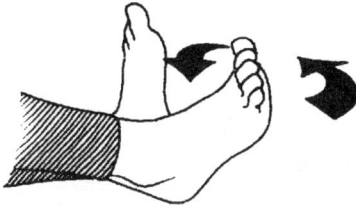

Exercise 1. To improve the circulation of blood in the legs. With your legs straight, make small circles with your feet.

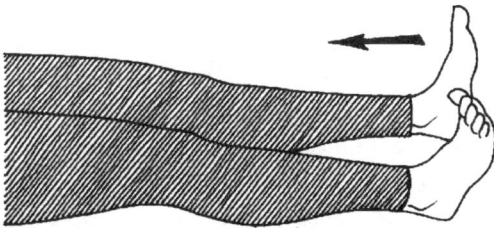

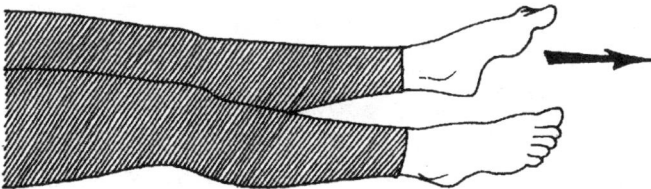

Exercise 2. To improve the circulation of blood in the legs. Keeping your heels on the bed or floor, raise and stretch your feet.

While you are immobile after your operation, you will probably be wearing anti-embolism stockings to improve the circulation of blood in your legs (see p. 51). However, you should also do the following exercises from the first post-operative day.

Sit on your bed, or on the floor, with your legs stretched out in front of you.

Exercise 1. Keeping your legs straight, make small circles with your feet.

Exercise 2. With your legs and heels on the bed, point your feet down and then pull them up towards you.

Exercise 3. Press the backs of your knees down onto the bed and then relax your legs.

Do each of these exercises ten times every 2 hours for at least 2 weeks after your operation – until you are walking as much as you were before it.

Coughing and sneezing

If you have had an abdominal hysterectomy, coughing, sneezing or vomiting may make your wound hurt during the first few days after your operation as these activities cause the muscles in the abdominal wall to tighten. Although coughing is unlikely to do any harm to your stitches, it will be less uncomfortable if you support your wound with your hands and bend both your knees to help reduce the tension in the muscles of your abdomen.

If lying in bed, bend your knees and put your feet flat on the bed while you support your wound. If sitting, lean slightly forward.

Getting out of bed

Getting out of bed may be difficult and possibly painful for a few days as the movement involved causes tightening of the abdominal muscles. The following method may be helpful.

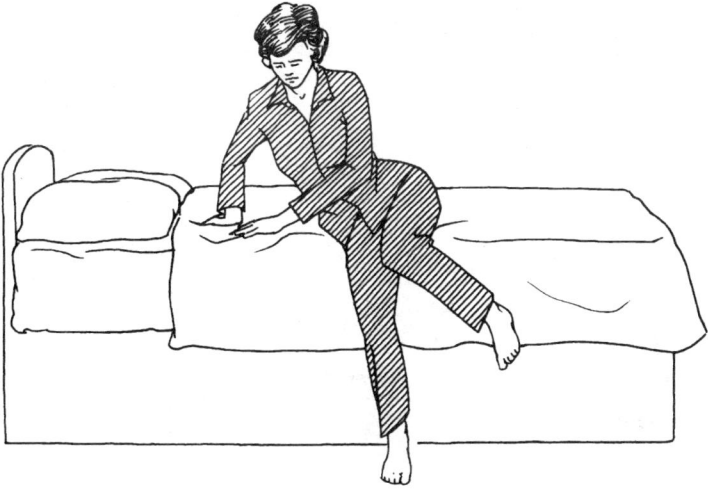

Getting out of bed. Once you have pushed yourself up from lying (as described in the text), you can gently lower your legs over the side of the bed.

1   Lie on your back and bend your knees up one at a time until your feet are flat on the bed.

2   Turn your head and shoulders to face the edge of the bed. With your knees together, roll on to your side.

3   Put your hands on the bed and use your arms to push yourself up into a sitting position, lowering your legs, one at a time, over the side of the bed until your feet touch the floor.

To get back into bed, follow the same guidelines but in reverse.

Lifting

All *heavy* lifting should be avoided for several weeks after a hysterectomy. This can be difficult for women with small children, but a child can be cuddled while you are sitting down,

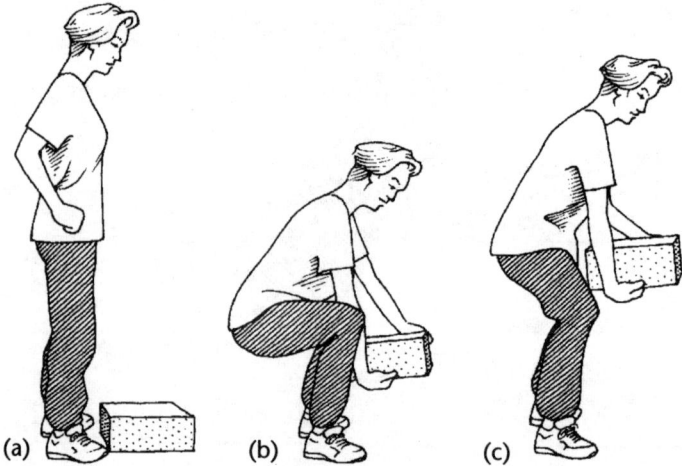

Lifting. The correct lifting technique is important at all times, but particularly so after an abdominal operation. (a) Stand close to the object, with your feet slightly apart and firmly on the ground. (b) Bend your knees (not your back) and grasp the object firmly in both hands. (c) Straighten your knees slowly until you are standing.

or with the child, if old enough, standing on a bed in front of you.

If you do have to lift anything, you should use the correct lifting technique described below. This is important at all times, not just following an operation.

1   Stand close to the object to be lifted, with your feet slightly apart and placed firmly on the floor.

2   Lower your body towards the object by bending your knees. Do *not* bend your back.

3   Grasp the object firmly in both hands, holding it close to you.

4   Slowly straighten your knees until you are standing.

5 Once you are upright, turn by moving your *feet*, not by twisting your back.

Reverse these steps to put an object down.

Posture

You may find the discomfort in your wound makes you slump forward, particularly when you are standing. You should try to avoid this as it will eventually lead to low back pain. Try to sit and stand with your back straight at all times – not with it sagging or arching backwards – as this will help to improve the tone of your abdominal muscles.

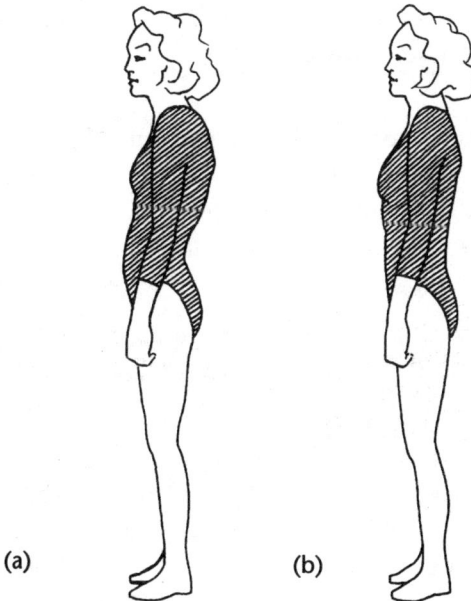

Posture. (a) Incorrect posture will eventually lead to low back pain. (b) Standing with your back straight will help to tighten your stomach muscles.

Other exercises

Once you feel able to start some gentle exercises – probably about a week after your hysterectomy – you should do them every day while lying on your bed or on the floor. If you have had any problems with the healing of your wound, or the wound is uncomfortable, you should wait a little longer before starting these exercises.

The exercises described here are to strengthen your abdominal muscles and the muscles in your pelvis which support your vagina and the openings from your bladder and rectum.

Exercise 1
Pull the muscles around your back passage up and in tightly and then tighten and lift your front passage. Hold these up as firmly as you can for 5 seconds and then let them go. Do this exercise five times, at least ten times a day.

Exercise 2
Lie on your back with one leg bent and one straight. Try to make the straight leg shorter by pulling it up at the hip. Then repeat the exercise with the other leg. Do this ten times with each leg. This exercise can also be done while standing.

Exercise 3
Lie on your back with both knees bent and your feet flat on the bed or floor. Press the middle of your back down and hold for 6 seconds before you relax. Repeat this exercise five times.

Exercise 4
Lie on your back with both knees bent and press the middle of your back down, keeping your knees together. Then twist from your waist to roll your knees over towards the bed or floor on one side. Then roll them to the other side, trying to get further each time until you are able to touch the bed with your knees. Repeat this in both directions five times.

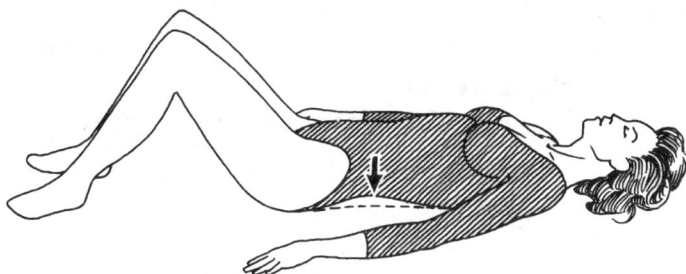

Exercise 3. To strengthen the muscles of the abdomen and pelvic floor. With both knees bent, press the middle of your back down onto the floor or bed.

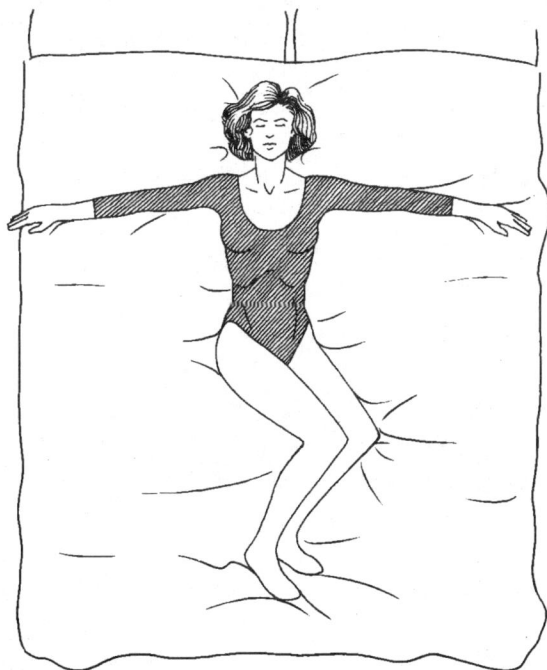

Exercise 4. To strengthen the muscles of the abdomen and pelvic floor. With both knees bent, twist from your waist to roll your knees towards the bed or floor.

Exercise 5

Lie on your back with both knees bent. Press the middle of your back down onto the bed, and lift your head and shoulders and reach your hands towards your knees.

If you do these exercises regularly, you should gradually begin to notice an improvement in the strength of your abdominal muscles. If the muscles of the pelvic floor are not strengthened after an operation of this sort (or after giving birth), incontinence can occur in later life as the muscles which control the openings to the bladder and rectum are too weak to hold back the flow of urine or the passage of faeces.

CHAPTER 11

Possible complications

All operations carry a small risk of complications such as deep vein thrombosis or chest infection. Precautions are taken to try to prevent complications such as these occurring, for example compression stockings are worn to assist the circulation of blood and help avoid the formation of blood clots in your legs while you are immobile.

Bruising is common after any type of surgery, and can be extensive, taking several days or sometimes weeks to fade. Although the sight of a severe bruise can be shocking, it is rarely a cause for concern.

Minor post-operative complications are fairly common, but serious ones are rare. At their 6-week post-operative check-up after a hysterectomy, most women say they feel much less tired and generally much better than they did before their operation.

Damage to the bladder or bowel
If, as occasionally happens, the bladder or bowel is damaged during surgery, for example by being pierced with a sharp surgical instrument, the damage will have to be surgically repaired. In the case of damage to the bladder, a catheter will have to be kept in place for 4 to 7 days, and antibiotics will be necessary to avoid an infection developing. Damage to the bowel will require a regime of 'nil by mouth', and fluids will have to be administered intravenously through a drip. Very rarely, damage is sufficiently severe to necessitate a colostomy – an operation to enable the faeces to be removed from the body into a colostomy bag without passing down the colon.

Complications after abdominal or vaginal hysterectomy

Short-term complications

There are certain general complications which can follow an abdominal or vaginal hysterectomy, both of which constitute major surgery.

Primary haemorrhage   Haemorrhage simply means bleeding. Although some bleeding is inevitable during any type of surgery, it can cause problems if heavy. Primary haemorrhage can occur at the time of the operation and, if severe, may require a blood transfusion.

Secondary haemorrhage   Secondary haemorrhage is bleeding which occurs after surgery and it can usually be dealt with by placing a pack in the vagina to absorb the blood, or by putting a pressure dressing on the abdominal wound. If blood loss is heavy, return to theatre or a blood transfusion may be necessary.

Once you have returned home, secondary haemorrhage, which can occur 1 to 2 weeks later, may be due to the release of blood from a haematoma that formed at the time of surgery or to an infection that has developed subsequently. Infection can usually be treated with antibiotics. Iron tablets may also be necessary if blood loss has been heavy. Only rarely is re-admission to hospital necessary for blood transfusion.

Seek advice from your GP or the hospital out-patients' department if you are at all concerned about bleeding, particularly if the loss is of bright red, and therefore fresh blood. If bleeding seems to be excessive, seek medical advice urgently.

Haematoma   A haematoma is a swelling composed of blood. It can occur if blood collects under the wound. Although wound haematomas usually resolve themselves – sometimes by discharging a gush of blood – they can be painful and lead to extensive bruising. **A vaginal haematoma** can develop if the blood collects at the top of the vagina, and this may make you feel generally unwell. The blood will either be absorbed or discharged.

Post-operative anaemia   Anaemia is normally treated with iron and depends on the haemoglobin level prior to surgery and on the amount of blood lost during the operation. Usually less than 1 pint (about 300 ml) of blood is lost during hysterectomy, but this varies depending on the size of the uterus and how mobile and easy it was to remove. Blood transfusion is occasionally necessary if more immediate treatment for anaemia is required.

Wound infection   Infection can occur in the cut in the vagina, and bacteria can pass from there into the abdominal cavity. Infection of the abdominal wound is also possible and, if it occurs, an **abscess** may form and the wound will become red, hard and tender, and may discharge pus. You may feel generally unwell, with fever and sweating. Abscesses can be treated with antibiotics, but are often best dealt with by release of the pus they contain.

Urinary infection   It is unusual not to be able to pass urine spontaneously within 48 to 72 hours after a hysterectomy, but if urinary retention does develop, a catheter may need to be passed into the bladder. An infection of the urinary tract may lead to a raised body temperature, pain when passing urine, frequent passage of urine, low back pain, or a general feeling of being unwell; or there may be no symptoms. If an infection is suspected, your urine may be tested to see if any infective organisms are present. Urinary infections can sometimes be cleared up by increasing the amount you drink, but treatment with antibiotics may be necessary, the type of antibiotic used depending on the strain of organism identified.

Paralytic ileus   This is a temporary paralysis of the bowels, causing distension of the abdomen, discomfort and vomiting if severe. Treatment involves being starved, with fluids being given through an intravenous drip until the condition resolves itself, normally within 24 hours but occasionally taking up to 3 to 4 days. Paralytic ileus is fairly common during the first 24 hours after surgery, particularly after abdominal hysterectomy, but is uncommon after this.

Constipation and altered bowel habit These are common, minor complications in the first week or two after a hysterectomy. A good healthy diet, exercise, and suppositories, if necessary, will help to resolve these problems.

Chest infection It is important to keep your lungs aerated post-operatively by doing deep breathing exercises (see p. 98). Chest infection can occur following anaesthesia for any type of operation, and is particularly common in smokers. Deep breathing is more difficult after abdominal hysterectomy because it may cause pain in the abdominal wound, and a physiotherapist will probably advise you about this while you are in hospital.

Deep vein thrombosis (DVT) Blood clots can form within the deep veins of the body, and deep vein thrombosis is relatively common following surgery. It occurs particularly in the calf veins of the leg or in the pelvis (where it cannot be seen). A clot, or **thrombus**, can pass through the heart and enter the arteries of the lungs, causing a sudden blockage known as pulmonary embolism. This can be life threatening and is the reason why compression stockings and heparin injections are necessary for patients who are not mobile. If a deep vein thrombosis is detected, it can be treated by a course of heparin and warfarin.

Pyrexia Pyrexia is simply fever, and can occur during the first 24 hours after the operation. If you have a high or persistent fever, a sample of your urine will be taken for analysis, and a doctor will listen to your chest, look for a leg DVT, and check your wound and abdomen for infection.

Longer-term complications

Abdominal and vaginal hysterectomies have similar long-term complications, some of which can also occur after laparoscopic hysterectomy. However, there may be numbness around the wound following an abdominal hysterectomy which can persist for several weeks.

Bladder function   There is no clear evidence concerning the effect of hysterectomy on long-term bladder function. Some women become incontinent or notice increased urgency and frequency after this operation. Alternatively, particularly for those who have had large fibroids in their uterus or prolapse of the womb, bladder function may seem to be improved.

None of these effects is surprising if you consider the need to move the bladder during the operation, and the possibility that its nerve or blood supply may be damaged.

Problems with bladder function may be due to the hysterectomy having revealed or exacerbated an abnormality that was there before. This possibility needs to be investigated by tests on the bladder; the problem can then be treated, if necessary, by medication or an operation.

Sexual function   Sexual function following hysterectomy is largely uninvestigated, although it would be fairly simple to obtain data by asking women about their experiences. The role of the cervix is not well understood in sexual intercourse.

Although it is possible that the vagina may be shortened during an abdominal hysterectomy, this is rare, and it normally returns to its original length. However, problems can occur if a repair of the vaginal walls was done at the same time, particularly a posterior repair, and many surgeons now try to avoid this.

Many women have a satisfactory sex life after having a hysterectomy; others complain that they do not feel quite the same. There is no medical reason why the vagina should not be as wet as it was before the operation.

If you do experience sexual or bladder function problems, you should tell your doctor. Help is available for both. Problems with sexual function may have a physical cause which your doctor can investigate and correct. However, psychological problems are not uncommon, and if the cause is not physical, your GP should be able to give you details of counsellors who may be able to help.

Complications after laparoscopically assisted hysterectomy

After laparoscopically assisted hysterectomy, deep vein thrombosis or chest infection is still possible, although these complications are far less common than after an abdominal or vaginal hysterectomy. Even wound infection can develop in the tiny wounds in the abdomen, although this is rare.

Paralytic ileus, and constipation do occur after laparoscopic hysterectomies, but they are rare complications. Haemorrhage and urinary tract infection are possible.

If there is substantial bleeding during laparoscopic surgery, the blood will obscure the area of operation, and the surgeon will have to resort to conventional abdominal surgery. The likelihood of this occurring will depend on your anatomy, the amount of disease present, the size of your uterus and how stuck it is, as well as on the experience of the surgeon.

As with other types of hysterectomy, any of the abdominal organs can be damaged during a laparoscopic operation and, if this happens, the abdomen will probably have to be opened as for conventional surgery and the affected organ will have to be repaired.

Laparoscopically assisted vaginal hysterectomy has not been routinely performed for sufficient time for its long-term effects on bladder and sexual function to have been assessed, but it does appear to be similar in these respects to an abdominal or vaginal hysterectomy.

Complications after endometrial resection

Following an endometrial resection, pregnancy is still possible and must be avoided as the placenta may be implanted abnormally leading to dangers for the woman and her baby.

Short-term complications

Because this is a short operation, and not painful, chest infections and deep vein thrombosis are unlikely post-operatively, as is paralytic ileus. There is, of course, no skin wound to be infected. However, urinary tract infection is possible if a bladder catheter has been used. Infection can also occur in the uterine cavity.

As with all types of hysterectomy, any organ can be damaged during an endometrial resection, and the surgeon will have the necessary skills to repair it should this happen.

The usual complications associated with anaesthesia can also occur (see p. 115).

Uterine perforation If the surgeon cuts or burns too deeply during an endometrial resection and the uterus is perforated, an exploratory operation called a **laparotomy** will have to be done to make sure that other vital structures such as the bladder or bowel have not been damaged. There is also a risk of haemorrhage from the uterus.

Laparotomy involves making a long incision in the abdomen so that the surgeon can examine the abdominal cavity, and if a laparotomy is carried out, the surgeon will probably also do a hysterectomy at the same time. It is therefore important to discuss with the surgeon before your operation what you would wish to be done should this situation arise. You should, however, always be prepared to accept hysterectomy if the surgeon thinks it is essential.

Bleeding from the uterus without perforation Some bleeding is normal after endometrial resection, but if this is very

113

heavy, the surgeon may deem it necessary to proceed straight to a hysterectomy. Alternatively, a catheter may be passed into the uterus to inflate it and put pressure on the blood vessels to stop them bleeding. The catheter will remain in place for about 4 to 6 hours post-operatively. In most cases, the bleeding will stop, but an overnight stay in hospital may be necessary for observation.

Other complications   Because fluid is used to irrigate the uterus during endometrial resection, a very careful check is kept on the amount that enters and leaves the body. If too much fluid is absorbed, it can lead to heart failure and intoxication syndrome (see p. 75). To avoid this, the surgeon will stop operating should more than 1 litre of glycine be unaccounted for. As long as this rule is followed by the surgeon, you are extremely unlikely to suffer these complications. It may mean that the operation has to be completed at a second attempt, but this is unlikely for any surgeon who has done a reasonable number of these procedures.

Longer-term complications

After endometrial resection, bladder function should be as normal. As the ovaries, cervix and nerves are still intact, sexual intercourse should also be unaffected.

Endometrial cancer   If, following an endometrial resection, bleeding stops and then recurs, you should consult your doctor. If parts of the endometrium are still present, it is possible for endometrial cancer to develop, and this will need to be investigated.

Pain   Rarely, if a small amount of endometrium is left behind after the operation, this will bleed at the time of menstruation each month. If the blood is unable to escape because the cervical canal is blocked by scar tissue, it will collect in the uterine cavity under pressure, and this tension in the wall of the womb will cause pain. This complication has only recently been recognised. It is usually managed by hysterectomy, or possibly by repeating the endometrial resection.

Risks and complications of general anaesthesia

Despite the tremendous advances in anaesthesia in recent years, there is always a small risk associated with the use of a general anaesthetic, and great care is taken to select the one which is most suitable for each patient.

If, as happens very rarely, the supply of oxygen to the brain is interrupted for some reason, brain damage, possibly with paralysis, or death can occur. It is important to understand and consider this risk, although it is a very small one: you are far more likely to be run over while crossing the road than to suffer any serious complication as a result of a general anaesthetic.

Minor complications of anaesthesia are a sore throat, due to the 'dry' anaesthetic gases used, or resulting from a tube being put down your throat to help you breathe. Coughs and chest infections can also occur, as well as muscle aches and pains caused by the muscle relaxants used. Muscle pain usually lasts no longer than 48 hours.

If a complication does arise

If you are at all concerned about anything that occurs during your recovery from your operation, contact your doctor, the consultant, or hospital ward for advice. If you leave a message with your consultant's secretary, the consultant will get in touch with you to discuss your problem.

Although the majority of complications are minor, it is always better to err on the safe side and to explain what has happened to a doctor, who can put your mind at rest or, if necessary, arrange for any appropriate treatment.

CHAPTER 12

Private care

There are various reasons why people choose to have their operations done privately. They may have private health insurance, or be covered by a private health scheme run by the company for which they work, or they may be able to pay for private care themselves. Whatever your situation, you will not find that the *standard* of medical care you receive in a private hospital is any different from that available on the National Health Service (NHS). However, you may prefer the privacy of a private hospital; or you may find the much-reduced waiting time to see a consultant, and to enter hospital for your operation, is more convenient for you. If you have a hysterectomy in an NHS hospital, you may rarely see the consultant, being examined by different doctors in the consultant's firm. At a private hospital, you will receive personal care from the consultant throughout your stay. The facilities at a private hospital are likely to be more like those of a good hotel, and will certainly include a private bathroom – a particular bonus for women who have had a hysterectomy.

The information given in other chapters in this book is equally relevant whichever system you choose. This chapter deals with those aspects of private health care which differ from those of the NHS.

Private health insurance

If the company you work for has a private health insurance scheme, your Company Secretary will be able to give you details, and should be able to tell you if the company insurance covers you for consultation with the surgeon, a D & C, a hysterectomy or endometrial resection.

If you have your own private health insurance, the insurance company will be able to tell you exactly what is covered by your particular policy, if this is not clear from the literature you already have.

There are different levels of health insurance, and you need to check your policy carefully to make sure you know what costs are covered. Most private hospitals have an administration officer who will check your policy for you if you are in any doubt. The staff at the hospital are likely to be very helpful and will try to sort out any problems and queries you have. But do read your policy carefully, and any information sent to you by the hospital, as unexpected charges, such as consultants' fees that you thought were covered by your insurance policy, could add up to quite a lot of money.

With some types of private health insurance, you will need to ask your GP to fill in a form stating that your operation is necessary and cannot be done in an NHS hospital within a certain time period due to long waiting lists. You will have to pay your GP for this service, which will cost a few pounds. This money is not redeemable from your insurers.

Fixed Price Care

You may be in the position of being able to pay to have your operation done privately. The Bookings Manager at a private hospital will be able to give you an idea of the cost involved. Some private hospitals run a service known as Fixed Price Care: a price can be quoted to you before you enter hospital which covers the cost of your operation and a variety of other hospitalisation costs. You should always ask to have the quotation in writing *before* you enter hospital, with a written note of everything it covers. At some hospitals, the fixed price will include accommodation, nursing, meals, drugs, dressings, operating theatre fees, X-rays etc.; at others only some of these are included. Once you have a quotation, you should not have to worry about any hidden costs that you had not accounted for. However, the price quoted to you by the hospital may not include the fees of the consultant surgeon or consultant anaesthetist, and you may have to ask your consultant for a note of these.

With Fixed Price Care, all the hospitalisation costs included by that particular hospital are covered should you need to stay longer than expected in hospital (usually up to a maximum of 28 days) as a direct result of complications arising from your original reason for admission. In other words, if you develop some problem while in hospital that is unrelated to the menstrual problems which led to your need for your operation, the price you have been quoted will not cover treatment to deal with this. If, on the other hand, you should have heavy bleeding post-operatively, or some other complication which makes your consultant decide to keep you in hospital for longer than originally planned, all the costs that arise from your stay and are included in the hospital's fixed price (again, with the possible exception of consultants' fees) will be covered. At some hospitals, the quoted price will also cover your treatment should you have to be re-admitted due to a complication related to your original operation and arising within a limited period of time after your discharge.

The only extra charges that you will have to pay to the hospital will probably include those for telephone calls, any alcohol if you have this with your meals, food provided for your visitors, personal laundry done by the hospital, hairdressing, and for any similar items such as you would have to pay for in a hotel. It is usually possible for a visitor to eat meals with you in your room, and for tea and snacks to be ordered for visitors during the day. (You will also have to pay these extra charges before you leave the hospital if you are being treated under private health insurance.)

It is important therefore that you ask in advance for *written confirmation* of the price you will have to pay for your stay in hospital and what is included in the quotation. If the hospital does not have a Fixed Price Care or similar system, make sure that all possible costs are listed.

Arranging the operation

Although the medical treatment you receive in a private hospital will be similar to that available at any NHS hospital, there are some basic differences between the two systems.

As with the NHS, you will have to be referred to a consultant by your GP. Most GPs have contacts with particular consultants (and private hospitals) to whom they tend to refer patients. If there is a private hospital you particularly want to go to, or a consultant you have some reason to prefer, you can ask your GP to make an appointment for you.

After your visit to your GP, you are unlikely to have to wait longer than a week or two before you see the consultant at an out-patient appointment. Your appointment may be at the private hospital where your operation is to be carried out, at an NHS hospital which has private wards, or at the consultant's private consulting rooms. Once the decision has been made to go ahead with surgery, you will probably be able to enter hospital at your convenience within another week or two.

You will receive confirmation of the date of your operation from the Bookings Manager of the hospital you are to attend. You will also probably be sent leaflets and any further relevant details of how to prepare for your admission to hospital. Do read these carefully, as knowing how your particular hospital organises things will help you to be prepared when you arrive for your operation. You will also be sent a **pre-admission form** to fill in and take with you when you are admitted.

If your operation is being paid for by insurance, you will be asked to take a completed insurance form with you when you are admitted to hospital. You should have been given some of these forms when you first took out your policy, but your insurance company will be able to supply the correct form if you have any problems. If you are covered by company insurance, the form will probably be filled in and given to you by your Company Secretary.

Admission to hospital

When you arrive at the hospital, the receptionist will contact the admissions department, and a ward receptionist will come to collect you. If you are paying for your stay in hospital yourself, you will probably be asked to pay your bill in advance at this stage if you have not already done so. Otherwise, you will be asked for your completed insurance form. The ward receptionist will take you to your room – probably a single or double room – and show you the facilities available there. You are likely to have a private bathroom, a television, and a telephone by your bed. The ward receptionist will explain hospital procedures to you, and will leave you to settle in.

A member of the nursing staff will then come to make a note of your medical details, in much the same way as described in Chapter 5. The main difference you are likely to notice if you have been treated in an NHS hospital before, is that this time there is much less waiting for all the routine hospital procedures to be dealt with. The nurse to patient ratio is higher in private hospitals and so someone is usually available to deal with the pre-operative procedures quite quickly.

Your consultant will deal with your medical care throughout your stay, will visit you before the operation, perform the operation (with the assistance of the anaesthetist and the operating staff), and visit you again when you are back in your own room. Trainees – whether doctors or nurses – do not work in private hospitals. The consultants are responsible for their own patients and supervise their care themselves. Most private hospitals now have resident medical officers – fully qualified, registered doctors who are available 24 hours a day to deal with any emergencies which may arise.

Preparing for your operation

When the time for your operation approaches, a porter and nurse will take you from your room to the anaesthetic room. In many private hospitals, you will not be moved from your bed onto a trolley until you have been anaesthetised; the bed itself will be wheeled from your room. Similarly, you will be transferred back from the trolley to your own bed in the recovery room while you are still asleep. You therefore go to sleep and wake up in your own hospital bed.

Your operation will be performed in the same way as described in Chapter 7. When you are fully awake, you will be taken back to your room to rest.

Discharge from hospital

When you are ready to be discharged from hospital, the ward receptionist will ask you to pay any outstanding charges not covered by the hospitalisation charge. You will be given any medical items you may need from the hospital pharmacy.

Differences and similarities

The main aim of the staff of any private hospital is the same as that in an NHS hospital – to make your stay as pleasant and as comfortable as possible. Because the staffing ratio is higher in private hospitals, more emphasis can be placed on privacy and comfort.

The consultant surgeons and anaesthetists almost always work in an NHS hospital as well as in a private hospital, so you will receive the same expertise and skill under both systems. However, in an NHS hospital you may not actually be operated on by the consultant surgeon who heads the surgical team, and, indeed, you may not see the consultant at all during your stay.

Private hospitals arrange their operating lists differently from NHS hospitals. The NHS hospitals have 'sessional bookings' for their operating theatres. This means a particular day is set aside at regular intervals for a specialist in one type of surgery to perform operations. In private hospitals, the consultants can book the use of an operating theatre (and the assistance of the staff who work in it) on any day, at any time that suits them. Therefore, your operation can take place privately with minimum delay, and at a time that is convenient to you and your consultant.

It is also possible, even if you are already on an NHS waiting list, to tell your GP or consultant at any time that you would like to change to private care. If the consultant you have already seen under the NHS does not have a private practice, you can ask to be put in touch with a consultant who *can* see you privately.

Summary

There are several reasons why, if they can, some women choose to have their operations done privately, either paid for by private health insurance or from their own pockets. Some find it much more convenient to be able to have a say in when their operation is to take place. The NHS, under which the majority of people are treated, naturally has longer waiting lists. Even a relatively major operation such as a hysterectomy is not an emergency, and therefore you will not be placed at the top of the waiting list for your operation to be done on the NHS. If time is an important factor for you, you may be happy to pay to have your operation done at a time that you find convenient.

Some people simply prefer the smaller, more intimate setting they are likely to find in a private hospital. Private hospitals rarely deal with accidents and emergency treatment; the operations carried out in them are normally planned, at least a day or two in advance. Therefore, they do not have the bustle of an NHS hospital which has to deal with emergency admissions as well as the routine admissions for non-emergency operations.

A private bathroom adjoining a single- or double-bedded room can also be an advantage after an operation like a hysterectomy, which involves post-operative vaginal bleeding. Bathroom facilities are usually modern and cheerful, and are close to hand and available whenever needed.

Questions and answers

The answers to most of the questions below can be found elsewhere in this book. However, you may find them helpful in compiling your own list of questions to ask your GP or consultant. It is useful to write down questions as they occur to you, and to take your list with you to your doctor's appointment. Most people find it difficult to remember the things they wanted to ask when they are trying to take in the information being given to them by their doctor.

The answers given here are general, and your GP or surgeon may have slightly different information to give you, depending on what happens at your particular hospital.

Do ask your GP, the hospital doctor who is in charge of your care, or a member of the nursing staff if there is anything you do not understand. No question is too trivial, particularly if it concerns something that is worrying you.

1. *The dissolvable stitches in my abdominal wound following a recent hysterectomy are still visible. Although I had a bath after the wound dressing was removed in hospital, my friend said I shouldn't allow the wound to get wet until the stitches have gone. Is this true?*

Although the wound should not be allowed to become sodden, it is all right for you to have a bath, drying the area around the wound carefully afterwards.

2. *My mother says I should not do anything for several weeks after my hysterectomy as I could cause internal damage if I do. I have young chil-*

dren and know it will be impossible to do nothing at all, and am therefore very worried about how I will manage. When will I be able to cook and clean and look after my children again?

It is sensible to be careful after a hysterectomy, but you should gradually increase your amount of activity and exercise to avoid developing blood clots in the deep veins of your legs and pelvis.

You will probably feel quite tired and weak for at least a few days after your operation, and will want to take things easy, but there is no medical reason why you should not do whatever you feel able to do. The important thing is not to lift or push anything *heavy* as this could burst the stitches in your wounds – either in the external abdominal wound if you have one, or in the internal wounds where your tissues have been cut and then stitched.

You will probably not feel strong enough to do any heavy housework for a few days, particularly if you have had an abdominal hysterectomy. Nor will you want to stand for long periods to prepare meals etc. If help is available to you, do take advantage of it until you feel a bit better. But do not be afraid to do the things you think you can manage. When you start to feel tired, or your abdomen begins to ache, stop and rest.

If you have to look after your children alone, try to organise activities for them that you can do sitting down when you need to. Even young children can be heavy, so try to avoid lifting them if you can.

If you have had a laparoscopic operation, you will begin to feel better after only a few days.

3.   I will have to make quite complicated arrangements for my family to be looked after while I am in hospital, and therefore need to know exactly how long it will be before I am home again.

The length of time spent in hospital after a hysterectomy varies, and will depend in part on the type of operation you are having, your age, general medical condition, and whether you develop any post-operative complications. After an abdominal hysterectomy, you may be in hospital for about 7 days. A vaginal or laparoscopically assisted vaginal hysterectomy will mean a shorter stay, probably 3 or 4 days. Your admissions letter should give you some idea, but it is probably best to err on the safe side and then to cancel your arrangements if you are able to leave hospital early.

4. I am very frightened at the prospect of having to have a general anaesthetic for my hysterectomy. Is there an alternative type of anaesthesia?

Many people have a fear of never waking up again after a general anaesthetic but, with the anaesthetics used today, this is very unlikely. However, do discuss your anxieties with the anaesthetist when you are visited by this doctor on the ward before your operation. It may be possible for you to have an epidural anaesthetic, a type of local anaesthetic which is injected into your back and numbs your lower body. If so, you will probably also be given something to make you sleep during the operation, so that you will not be aware of what is happening. However, most surgeons prefer to do hysterectomies with patients under general anaesthesia as the operation is a major one. Epidurals are therefore not commonly used, unless there is a medical reason, such as a serious chest complaint, which makes a general anaesthetic inadvisable.

5. I had a hysterectomy 6 months ago, but still find sex difficult and uncomfortable. Is there anything I can do?

Although some doctors believe that a hysterectomy has no effect on sexual intercourse, the experience of many women suggests that it can do so. Your vagina may be drier than before your operation, and you may find that using a lubricating jelly, available from the chemist, will help. The situation will probably improve in time, but do ask your doctor's advice if you are concerned.

6. My husband wants to start having sex again, 6 weeks after my hysterectomy, but I am still afraid of it doing some damage. Should we wait a bit longer?

The longer you wait before starting sexual intercourse again, the more anxious you are likely to feel about it. There are stitches in the wound at the top of your vagina which will take a few weeks to heal, but by 6 weeks after your operation, gentle intercourse is very unlikely to do any damage.

7. Will sex still feel the same for my partner when we resume it after my hysterectomy?

This will partly depend on the size of your partner's penis, and on how vigorous his love-making. Although your cervix has been removed and your partner will no longer be able to feel it, this is not likely to affect his overall enjoyment of sex. The tightness of your vaginal opening will not have altered, and it is this, together with your response to him, that will govern his pleasure.

8. I had a hysterectomy 6 weeks ago, and my bowels are still not working properly. I go days at a time without a bowel motion, and when I do have one it is painful and difficult. I was told that it can take a while for your bowels to work normally again, but how long should I let this continue? My GP gave me a prescription for laxatives, but these have had no effect.

There is unlikely to be anything to worry about, unless you are vomiting or bleeding when you try to have a bowel motion. Some people's bowels take longer than others to get back into proper working order, and they may never be the same as they were before your operation. It is important to eat a high-fibre diet, containing brown bread and bran etc., and to get plenty of exercise. If you are sure you are eating properly, and are getting enough exercise, your GP may want to investigate this further. Do ask your doctor's advice if you are concerned.

9. I have been at home for 3 days after having a hysterectomy and still have a discharge. Is this normal?

It is normal to get some sort of discharge after a hysterectomy, and this will probably be a pink, watery fluid, which may continue for a few weeks. If the discharge is thick, and creamy white or smells unpleasant, you should make an appointment at your doctor's surgery so that a swab can be taken for examination. This type of discharge may be due to an infection, which can be easily treated.

10. Following an abdominal hysterectomy, my wound is healing well but my stomach feels very tender and bruised, although there is no bruising visible. Is this all right?

You will have had several layers of stitching inside your abdomen to close the cuts made in the muscle wall, and these internal wounds will take some time to heal. A hysterectomy also involves the surgeon handling your bladder and rectum to move them out of the way so that the uterus can be removed. Therefore there is bound to be bruising internally.

It may be up to 4 months before all the tenderness and bruised feelings disappear, and parts of your abdomen may feel slightly tender for longer.

11. I am 42 and due to have a hysterectomy and removal of both my ovaries. Will I have to have HRT and, if so, why and for how long?

It is advisable to have HRT until well after your menopause would have occurred, unless your operation was to treat cancer, in which case you will have to discuss this with your doctor.

Some doctors advise women to continue with HRT for the rest of their lives; others recommend it for 10 years. Many women are currently having HRT in their seventies and eighties, and many have been having it for 30 years or more.

Women's bones start to crumble long before their menopause, and by the age of 60, 1 in 10 women not having HRT will have broken a bone, such as a wrist, ankle or rib, in a trivial accident. Over the age of 70, 1 in 4 women not on HRT will have broken a bone, in many cases a hip bone, and 1 in 4 of these will die as a direct result; many more will be permanently disabled to some degree. Hormone replacement therapy prevents the gradual loss of bone and thus helps to avoid these risks. Therefore many doctors think that combined HRT, with oestrogen and progestogen, should start well before the menopause, as the loss of calcium which causes the bones to become brittle begins in a woman's forties.

Hormone replacement therapy also has a protective effect on the circulation; women not having this treatment are as likely as men to suffer a heart attack, and are also at increased risk of having a stroke. Leg ulcers due to poor blood circulation are another problem which is reduced by HRT. Oestrogen helps prevent the skin from thinning, which again provides some protection against the leg ulcers that can otherwise result from trivial knocks and bangs, and which may require daily dressing and treatment for months or years. HRT also helps the skin in the vagina retain its moisture.

Most women having HRT *feel* better than they do without it, and find that they have increased energy and enjoyment of life.

It is the progestogen part of combined HRT which tends to cause any side-effects experienced, and as replacement of this hormone is only necessary to prevent cancer of the womb, oestrogen alone will be enough after a hysterectomy.

12. I am due to have a hysterectomy but my ovaries are not being removed. How will they be supported in my body when they are no longer attached to my uterus?

The ovaries are not supported by the uterus. They are attached to the side walls of the pelvis by ligaments which remain in place after the uterus has been removed.

13. When will I be back to normal after my hysterectomy?

The answer to this question depends on various factors: your age, your state of health before your operation, what is 'normal' for you, and possibly on how keen you are to get going again. If, for example, you do a job which involves strenuous physical activity or using heavy machinery, such as an electric floor polisher, it may be 4 months or so before you are able to work normally again. If you are well-motivated and your work is less physically demanding, you may be able to start again within 4 to 6 weeks.

Young women, whose muscles are stronger and more elastic, often recover quite quickly. The muscles of older women are likely to take longer to heal and to regain their strength.

If you had very heavy periods and were constantly tired before your operation, or if you suffered severe period pains, you may be surprised at how much better you feel within a couple of months.

Different women recover at different rates, and the recovery time is likely to be shorter following a vaginal or laparoscopic hysterectomy, but you can probably expect to return to your normal level of activity within 6 to 12 weeks.

14. How much pain will I have after my hysterectomy?

Some women have very little pain after a hysterectomy, some-times only for a couple of days, after which they suffer slight dis-comfort for a week or so. Others find the operation painful, and need to take pain-killing tablets for a couple of weeks. Many women find that the wind they have after a hysterectomy is more painful than the wounds themselves, but this should stop within a few days.

Although most operations are painful to some extent, there is really no need for anyone to suffer severe pain after an opera-tion, and you should ask a nurse or doctor for more effective pain relief if necessary.

15. I would like my husband to come with me to talk to the consultant when we discuss the possibility of my having a hysterectomy. Do you think the consultant will object to this?

The consultant is very unlikely to object to you taking someone with you to your appointment. Indeed, it is often a good idea to do so if you think you may not absorb all that is told to you. If the consultant seems brusque, it will be because the clinics are very busy, and there is considerable pressure and lack of time. It is very unlikely to be because the consultant is annoyed with you.

16. A lump has appeared under my wound and it seems to be getting big-ger. What should I do?

Although this is unlikely to be anything to worry about, it is advisable to make an appointment to see your GP. The lump is probably a haematoma, which is a swelling composed of blood that has been unable to escape through your wound. Although this may be painful, it is likely to resolve itself within a few days. Haematomas usually develop within about 48 hours post-opera-tively.

If your wound is red, hard and painful, and is discharging pus, it may be infected, and the pus may have collected in an abscess. An abscess can develop up to 2 weeks after an operation, and may need to be treated with antibiotics and release of the pus.

17. *During a recent D & C operation, fibroids were found on my uterus. Will I have to have a hysterectomy or is there an alternative treatment? I am 35, and may want to have another child in the future.*

Fibroids are swellings of muscle which are quite common in the uterus, and in most cases do not cause any ill-effects. Small, symptomless fibroids do not require treatment. Larger ones can, however, lead to heavy periods and in some cases to fertility problems. Drugs are available which will shrink the fibroids, but this is only a temporary treatment, and they will grow again within a few months. An operation may be possible to remove the fibroids while retaining your womb, and if so, you may have to take drugs for a while beforehand to shrink the fibroids and make them easier to remove. Your consultant will be able to discuss this with you.

18. *I had a hysterectomy a couple of months ago, and although I feel physically much better, I still feel occasionally weepy and rather depressed. Will this ever pass?*

Your doctor may suggest you start HRT, and the oestrogen should help to make you feel better and more energetic. Although it is not uncommon for women to feel depressed for a while after a hysterectomy, it is not your uterus that makes you a woman, so losing it should not make you less of one. Your femininity is locked into every part of your being, and does not just depend on your ability to have children. Many women cannot, or do not wish to, have children for a variety of reasons, and most feel secure in their womanliness. It is quite natural to feel saddened at the end of your child-bearing years, when you no longer have the choice about whether or not to have children, but this would have happened at your menopause anyway.

Most large cities have a hysterectomy support group, and you may find it helpful and comforting to talk to women who have gone through the same emotional upheaval as you are going through. Your GP or hospital should be able to give you details of a support group in your area.

19. I am due to have an endometrial ablation. If this operation does not resolve my heavy, painful periods, will I be able to have a hysterectomy?

There should be no reason why you cannot have a hysterectomy if endometrial ablation fails to solve your menstrual problems. Although the periods of 90% of women are less heavy or stop altogether once the endometrial lining of the womb has been removed, about 10% subsequently require a hysterectomy.

20. Is it possible for me to get pregnant after having an endometrial resection?

Your ovaries will remain in place after your operation and will continue to release an egg each month. Your periods may continue, although if they do they will probably be much lighter than before. It is therefore still possible for you to conceive, and you should use some form of contraception until your menopause. A pregnancy could be dangerous, both for you and for your baby.

21. Do I need to have cervical smears now that I have had an endometrial resection, and would I need to have them if I went on to have a hysterectomy?

Endometrial resection does not reduce your risk of developing cancer of the cervix, womb or uterus, as these are still in place. You should therefore continue to have regular cervical smears to detect any pre-cancerous abnormalities in your cervix. As it is unlikely that all the endometrium has been removed, it is also still possible to develop endometrial cancer.

If you go on to have a hysterectomy, your cervix and womb will be removed and, if your cervical smears have always been normal, there will be no need to continue them. However, if your smears have ever shown any abnormality, your doctor will probably suggest that you continue to have them, and will discuss this with you.

22. What type of hormone replacement therapy will I need after I have had an endometrial resection?

There will probably be some pockets of endometrium left in your uterus following endometrial resection and, as oestrogen alone may cause endometrial cancer, you should have a combined form of HRT containing both oestrogen and progestogen.

23. Having had a hysterectomy, how will I know when I am becoming post-menopausal?

You may have no menopausal symptoms at all, or you may experience the common symptoms of hot flushes, sweats, mood changes and tiredness. These are caused by the fall in the level of the female hormones produced by the ovaries, and removal of the uterus alone will not affect them. If the ovaries are removed, the production of these hormones is stopped suddenly, and severe menopausal symptoms can then occur for a few weeks unless hormone replacement therapy is taken. If your ovaries have been retained, they will cease to function around the time you could have expected to have your menopause – usually around the age of 50 – and you may get menopausal symptoms. You should consider HRT in any case to protect you against osteoporosis and to improve any symptoms you may have.

Case histories

The case histories which follow are not intended to make any specific point. They have been chosen at random as examples of the experiences of different women, and are included simply to illustrate the reality of having a hysterectomy or endometrial resection for these women. It should also be remembered that some women's menstrual problems can be treated effectively by drugs, without the need for any type of surgery.

CASE 1

Lynne is 33, and the mother of two young children.

When she began to have painful periods and a deep pain with sexual intercourse, her GP arranged for her to see a consultant. After discussion with the consultant, Lynne began a course of drug treatment, but this had little effect, and a few months later she had an exploratory laparoscopic operation which showed that she had endometriosis.

After a few months, Lynne was admitted to hospital for a total abdominal hysterectomy and the removal of both her ovaries. For the first 3 days after her operation, she used a patient-controlled pump to administer a pain-killing drug as and when she needed it. After this, she was given paracetamol tablets to help control the discomfort which was mainly caused by severe wind and which continued for several days.

When Lynne returned home, 7 days after her operation, she was looked after by her husband. She felt quite weak and tired for a few days, but was able to make herself cups of coffee and potter around the house, gradually beginning to feel better and to increase the amount she could do. Her wound healed well, becoming barely visible as her pubic hair regrew.

As Lynne had some residual endometriosis, at her 6-week check-up the consultant started her on a course of the contraceptive pill.

Although Lynne was very pleased to be rid of the period pains she had come to dread, she still found sexual intercourse painful after her operation, and as she felt that this could be psychologically based, her consultant arranged for her to talk to a sex therapist.

CASE 2

Caroline is an apparently healthy, slim, 48-year-old. She has two children, and has had several miscarriages.

About 2 years before her operation, Caroline began to have heavy, painful periods and her GP referred her to a consultant. She had a D & C, followed about 3 months later by an abdominal hysterectomy and the removal of both her ovaries. She does not remember much about the time immediately after her operation as she was rather confused when she came round from the anaesthetic.

The day after her hysterectomy, Caroline collapsed on the ward and was given a blood transfusion. She was then returned to the operating theatre for investigations to see if she was bleeding. There was no bleeding, but Caroline was found to be in heart failure. The next thing she remembers is waking up in the intensive care ward, having suffered a heart attack. She remained in intensive care for a week, and then spent a further week on a coronary ward, after which, as she was having difficulty sleeping, she was allowed to return home to recuperate.

She was very weak for several days, and continued to find sleeping difficult. Although her abdominal wound was only mildly uncomfortable, she felt bruised and battered.

An appointment was made for her to have some cardiac tests a couple of months after her operation.

Caroline and her family have been shocked and distressed by her experiences, and she finds the memory of what happened very upsetting. However, once she was over the initial shock, she began to appreciate the fact that she will no longer have to put up with the painful periods she had before her hysterectomy. **Note**. Although serious complications such as Caroline's do occur, for about 1 woman in 1000, they are rare, and her traumatic experience should be viewed in context. It is likely that she had an existing heart problem, which was exacerbated by the physical stress of her operation.

CASE 3

Sheila is 42 and has three daughters aged between 16 and 22.

At the age of 38, she had a coil fitted, after which her periods became much heavier, and she began to feel constantly tired. A blood test done by her GP showed no sign of anaemia. However, as she was finding her heavy periods difficult to cope with, she was referred to a consultant who suggested that the coil could be the cause of the problem. Sheila agreed to have it removed and to be sterilised at the same time.

As she felt sick when she awoke from the anaesthetic after the sterilisation and removal of her coil, she stayed in hospital overnight. She had only moderate post-operative discomfort, and returned to her work as a cleaner about 3 weeks later.

It was discovered during this operation that Sheila had fibroids in her womb. Unfortunately, her heavy periods continued and were not improved by the various drugs prescribed by the consultant, who then suggested a hysterectomy. With the prospect of possibly a further 10 years of difficult periods to put up with until her menopause, Sheila felt that this was her only real option. She was admitted to hospital a couple of months later for an abdominal hysterectomy.

Sheila had been anxious about having a general anaesthetic, but did not suffer from nausea or vomiting after her operation. She was given pain-killing injections for a couple of days post-operatively, as well as injections of heparin. After this, regular analgesic tablets helped to take the edge off her pain, which was mostly due to wind and which continued for about 4 days before easing off and recurring only occasionally for another week. Sheila had vaginal bleeding for a couple of days, and slight spotting for a few more. She was in hospital for 5 days after her operation, and the stitches were removed from her abdominal wound on the day before she went home.

Once at home, she had only slight discomfort and, although she felt tired and weak to begin with, was able to potter about the house, making tea and tidying up. Two weeks after her operation, she was able to go shopping with her family.

By the time she had her check-up at the hospital, about 8 weeks after her operation, Sheila's wound was healing well, but she was having only irregular bowel motions which, when they did occur, were difficult and painful. Her GP had given her a laxative, but this had had no effect. However, Sheila was very pleased with the results of her operation.

A couple of weeks later, she returned to her work as a cleaner and was able to do most of her jobs except using the electric floor polisher, which was heavy and made her abdomen ache.

CASE 4

Theresa is 27 and has four children aged between 2 and 8 years.

After her youngest child was born, her periods became painful and heavy. The tablets her GP prescribed had no effect, and Theresa asked about the possibility of having a hysterectomy. Her doctor suggested she have an endometrial resection, but as it would not guarantee an end to her periods, she opted for the hysterectomy.

About 2 months later, she saw a consultant and was admitted to hospital within 6 weeks for a laparoscopically assisted vaginal hysterectomy. As her ovaries could be expected to continue to function normally for several years, these were not removed.

Theresa had regular pain-killing injections for about 24 hours post-operatively. Her bladder functioned normally by the evening after her operation, and the following afternoon she was able to go home. She still felt drowsy and found walking quite painful.

Once at home, she went to bed, where she remained for a couple of days while her husband and other members of their family cared for the children and did the housework. She was a bit alarmed when she had a gush of blood from one of her small wounds, but the bleeding soon stopped.

Four days after her operation, Theresa went out with her husband, and a few days later she was able to do light housework and look after her family. She felt more or less back to normal within about 4 weeks.

Although she found the first few post-operative days more painful than she had expected, Theresa recovered from her hysterectomy quite quickly, and is very glad to have had it done.

CASE 5

Marilyn is 51 and has two daughters.

At the post-natal check-up after her second child was born – 19 years ago – the doctor noticed that she had a small prolapse of her womb. Regular exercises to strengthen the muscles in her pelvic floor seemed to help, and the prolapse caused her little trouble for several years. However, her womb did gradually prolapse further, and about 14 years later Marilyn's GP suggested something should be done about it. Unfortunately, the doctor she saw at the hospital was unhelpful, and although the prolapsed womb had started to cause Marilyn considerable discomfort, and pains in her legs when she walked any distance, he felt she would have to put up with it. Marilyn was so embarrassed by this encounter that she refused her GP's offer to arrange an appointment with another consultant.

About 4 years later, with a persistent vaginal infection, increasing discomfort, and very heavy periods, she had begun to find the prolapse difficult to cope with. Sitting down for an hour or so, having pushed her womb back up her vagina, would give her about half an hour of comfort, after which the womb would drop again and the discomfort would return. She therefore agreed to see another consultant, who was more sympathetic, and who suggested something should be done fairly quickly.

A couple of months later, Marilyn had a vaginal hysterectomy and the walls of her vagina were repaired. She was in hospital for only 3 days after her operation and had little post-operative pain, needing pain-killing injections for the first day, but thereafter only paracetamol. When she awoke from the anaesthetic, she was given injections to try to control frequent vomiting which lasted for several hours.

The bladder catheter which had been inserted during the operation was removed painlessly after a couple of days, and

Marilyn was able to pass urine soon afterwards. She had her first bowel motion before she went home, on the morning of the third post-operative day.

She felt weak and quite tired for a few days after she got home, and stayed in bed for a while each morning. By 2 weeks post-operatively, she was beginning to feel much better, and a week later her light, watery vaginal bleeding had stopped.

By the time of her check-up 6 weeks after her operation, she had made a good recovery, and was glad to have had the hysterectomy, only regretting that she put up with so many years of discomfort.

CASE 6

Katy is 40 and has two children, aged 3 and 8 years.

A couple of years after her younger child was born, she began to have difficulty inserting tampons. At about the same time, she started going to physiotherapy sessions and practising pelvic floor exercises as urine had begun to leak when she sneezed or coughed. Although the exercises did improve her bladder control, the problem with the tampons increased, until she was no longer able to use them and had to stop going swimming with her children when she had her periods. Her GP referred her to a consultant, whom she saw as a private patient to avoid having to wait for an appointment.

The consultant told Katy that her womb had prolapsed into her vagina, and offered her two alternative treatments. If she wanted to have more children, she could use a ring which she would have to insert into her vagina to help support the womb, taking it out before sexual intercourse. If she did not want any more children, she could have a hysterectomy, which, as the consultant pointed out, would probably be necessary eventually.

After talking to her husband and to her GP, Katy decided to

have the hysterectomy, which was done privately so that she could choose a convenient time to enter hospital. Although she was not suffering pain – only occasional discomfort during her periods – she had always had heavy periods, lasting about 7 days, and felt that it would be a relief not to have to put up with them any more.

Having gathered as much information as possible about her forthcoming operation, Katy was well prepared when she was admitted to hospital. She left hospital 5 days after having a vaginal hysterectomy, feeling quite rested. She only needed pain-killing injections during the first post-operative night, and took tablets for about a week.

After she had been home for a few days, Katy's husband had to return to work and, apart from arranging for someone to take her children to and from school and nursery, she was able to manage alone after the first week.

A couple of weeks after leaving hospital, she was able to go shopping, leaving her younger child with her husband as she did not feel she would be able to lift her or run after her should the need arise. Two weeks later, she was back to normal, cooking, doing the housework and driving, and by 5 weeks after her operation she was able to take up her hobby of horseriding again.

Case 7

Rachel is 41, with two sons aged 16 and 18.

Although she has always had heavy, painful and irregular periods, lasting several days, when they began to get even worse, and she had to use plastic pads to avoid soiling her sheets and chairs, she went to her GP.

Having taken a course of tablets for 3 months, with no improvement, Rachel underwent a laparoscopic investigation which showed fibroids on her womb. She was referred to a consultant, who suggested she have an endometrial resection preceded by a course of injections to shrink the lining of the womb.

Rachel was in hospital overnight following her operation, suffered no pain, and was back to normal after less than a week.

Her periods then settled into a regular pattern, occurring approximately every 4 weeks and lasting about 4 days, with only light menstrual bleeding and little accompanying pain.

Before her operation, Rachel had been taking evening primrose oil for some time to try to control the symptoms of premenstrual tension (PMT) which were always severe and sometimes brought her to the brink of violence. These symptoms were also much improved following surgery.

Medical terms

Abdomen/Abdominal cavity The body cavity between the diaphragm and the floor of the pelvis which contains the digestive organs – the stomach and intestines.

Abdominal hysterectomy The surgical removal of the uterus via an incision made in the abdominal wall.

Abscess A pus-filled cavity which has developed as a result of the disintegration of tissue.

Absorbable suture/stitches Stitches which are made of a material which is able to dissolve in the tissues, such as catgut or the synthetic fibre, Vicryl. Absorbable sutures do not need to be removed.

Adhesion The joining together of parts of the body which are normally separate.

Allergy An over-sensitivity to a particular substance which causes the body to react against it. The **allergic reaction** may be mild, such as an itchy rash, or it may be more severe, involving fainting, wheezing, vomiting or loss of consciousness. Your doctor should be told about any allergies you have so that they can be added to your medical records.

Amenorrhoea The absence of menstrual bleeding due to hormonal imbalance, physical or mental stress, or disease. The most common causes are pregnancy and hysterectomy.

Anaemia A condition of the blood in which there is a reduction in the number and quality of the red blood cells and/or a reduction in the amount of haemoglobin normally present. Anaemia can cause tiredness and pallor, and severe cases may have to be treated by blood transfusion, although iron medication is often sufficient.

Anaesthetic A drug used to cause loss of sensation or feeling in part of the body.

Analgesia The process by which pain is blocked, involving the use of pain-killing drugs.

Analgesic A drug which blocks sensations of pain; a painkiller.

Anovulatory bleeding Bleeding which may be cyclical but which occurs when a follicle ripens but fails to release an ovum.

Anteverted uterus The more usual orientation of the uterus, the tip of which bends forwards over the top of the bladder.

Antibiotic A substance which kills or prevents the reproduction of bacteria.

Anticoagulant A substance which reduces blood clotting, for example heparin and warfarin.

Anti-embolism stockings/Compression stockings/Thrombo-embolic deterrent stockings Stockings worn by patients during an operation to help prevent blood clots forming in the deep veins of the legs. The stockings work by assisting the circulation of the blood within the veins of the legs.

Anti-emetic A drug which helps to stop you vomiting or feeling sick.

Anti-fibrinolytic A substance which prevents the blood from forming clots.

Bilateral oophorectomy The surgical removal of both ovaries.

Biopsy The removal of a small piece of tissue from the body, usually for the purpose of diagnosis.

Birth canal The canal formed by the cervix and vagina through which a baby is born.

Blood clot A solidified mass of blood formed by its coagulation.

Blood transfusion The administration of whole blood or specific constituents of the blood into the body's blood vessels, usually via a vein in the arm. Blood may have to be transfused if large amounts are lost during an operation or if a specific factor is lacking from the patient's own blood.

Bronchitis   Inflammation of the lining of the bronchi, or air passages.

Caesarean section   Delivery of a fetus through an incision made in the mother's abdominal wall and in the wall of her uterus.

Cancer   A malignant growth caused by the uncontrolled multiplication of cells which, if left untreated, will eventually invade nearby areas of the body, and spread to distant parts.

Cannula   A very fine tube or needle which is inserted into a vein, usually in the back of the hand. Cannulas are used to introduce or remove fluids from the body, and to administer drugs such as anaesthetics. They are usually made of flexible plastic, but can be glass or metal. A common variety is the butterfly cannula.

Catheter   A thin tube used to withdraw or introduce fluid into the body. Bladder catheters are inserted into the bladder to drain the urine from it.

Cautery/Cauterisation   The process used to control bleeding or to destroy tissue during an operation, e.g. the endometrium is cauterised in endometrial ablation. (See also **Electrocautery**.)

Cervical smear test   The removal of a small sample of cells from the cervix of the uterus for examination under a microscope. The cells are scraped from the cervix using a specially shaped wooden spatula. The test is done to detect early precancerous cell changes which identify women at high risk of developing cervical cancer.

Cervix   The lower part of the uterus where it protrudes into the vagina.

Clitoris   A small external female genital organ which is similar to the penis in the male.

Coil   A plastic contraceptive device, with or without a copper wire coiled around the stem, which is inserted into the uterine cavity.

Complication   A condition which occurs as a result of another disease or treatment, e.g. venous thrombosis following a hysterectomy.

Compression stockings   See Anti-embolism stockings

Conception   The fertilisation of an ovum by a sperm.

Consent form   A form which patients must sign before surgery to confirm that their treatment has been explained to them, and that they understand what is to take place and have given their permission for the operation and anaesthesia.

Constipation   A condition in which opening of the bowels is difficult and infrequent.

Consultant   An experienced and fully trained doctor who specialises in a particular type of medicine.

Contraceptive   A drug or device which is used to prevent pregnancy.

Corpus   The body (of the uterus).

Corpus luteum   The yellow body which remains after an ovarian follicle has ruptured and released its ovum. It produces the hormone progesterone.

Cystectomy   An operation to remove a cyst.

Day-case surgery   An operation carried out on a patient who is in hospital for one day only, with no overnight stay.

Deep vein thrombosis (DVT)   A blood clot in the deep veins of the body, normally in the legs or pelvis.

Diarrhoea   The frequent passage of liquid stools.

Dilatation and curettage (D & C)   An operation to dilate the cervical canal in order to allow a sample of endometrium to be scraped out.

Discharge letter   A letter given to patients as they leave hospital which gives details of their treatment and any other information of which their family doctor should be aware.

Dissection   The separation or division of tissues or organs during a surgical operation.

Diuretic   A drug which increases the amount of urine produced.

Drain   A device which provides a channel for the passage of body fluids, often used to release discharge from a wound.

Drip   A device which allows fluid to be introduced into the body from a container connected to a tube. The fluid enters the body via a needle or cannula.

Dysfunctional uterine bleeding   Any abnormal menstrual bleeding which is heavier or less regular than usual and for which no cause has been identified.

Dyspareunia   Pain felt during sexual intercourse.

Dysmenorrhoea   Pain in the back or lower abdomen occurring during or around the time of menstruation. It is also commonly felt in the front of the thighs.

Electrocardiogram (ECG)   A record of the activity of the heart as a series of electrical wave patterns produced as the muscles in the heart beat.

Electrocardiography   The process by which an electro-cardiogram is recorded. Electrodes are taped to the skin over the heart and detect the electrical activity of the heart muscle.

Electrocautery   Cautery using an electric current to heat the tip of an instrument. The instrument can be applied to the ends of blood vessels to stop them bleeding, or can be used to remove the endometrium from the uterus.

Embolism   The sudden blocking of a blood vessel, usually caused by a blood clot or air bubble.

Embolus   (plural: **emboli**) A blood clot, or an air bubble, which blocks a blood vessel.

Emphysema   A condition in which the air sacs in the lungs are enlarged. The permanent expansion of the chest makes it difficult to take deep breaths, and causes shortness of breath. The most common cause is smoking.

Endometrial ablation   The destruction of the endometrium by electrical burning. See also **Endometrial resection**.

Endometrial biopsy   The surgical removal of a sample of tissue from the endometrium which is examined under a microscope to aid diagnosis.

Endometrial resection   The surgical removal of the endometrium from the uterus.

Endometriosis   The presence of pieces of endometrial tissue in places other than within the uterus, for example on the ovaries, and around the gut and external surface of the uterus.

Endometrium   The vascular layer lining the uterus, part of which is shed during menstruation.

Epidural anaesthetic   A local anaesthetic which is injected into the space around the spinal cord and numbs the back, legs and lower abdomen.

Epimenorrhoea   Normal bleeding, i.e. not unusually heavy or light, which occurs at abnormally short intervals.

Faeces   The undigested remains of food and other waste matter which is discharged from the rectum.

Fallopian tube   One of the two tubes through which ova pass on their way from the ovaries to the uterus.

Fertilisation   The union of an ovum and sperm to form an embryo.

Fetus   A developing embryo. (Also spelt **foetus**)

Fibroid   A localised, benign growth of the muscular tissue that forms the wall of the uterus.

Field block   Injection of an anaesthetic around the site of an operation. Nerves follow a predictable path, and can be blocked in specific areas, or 'fields', near the operation site.

Fixed Price Care   A system used by some private hospitals in which a fixed price is given for a particular operation and at least some of the hospitalisation costs it will involve.

Follicle   See **Ovarian follicle**

Follicle-stimulating hormone (FSH)   A hormone which stimulates the production of ovarian follicles. It is produced by the pituitary gland at the base of the brain.

Fornix   The part of the vagina into which the cervix protrudes.

Fundus   The part of the body of the uterus above the connections of the fallopian tubes.

General anaesthetic   A drug which induces sleep so that there is no sensation in any part of the body.

Granulation tissue   A mass of inflammatory tissue which may form where a wound is healing. It is bright red and bleeds easily when touched. The tissue is moist, and does not heal over quickly with skin.

Gynaecologist   A doctor who deals with the diagnosis and treatment of diseases affecting women.

Haematoma   A blood-filled swelling. Haematomas can form after surgery if a blood vessel continues to bleed. When the blood is spread in the tissues it appears as a bruise.

Haemoglobin   A protein within the red blood cells which carries molecules of oxygen and is involved in the process of respiration.

Haemorrhage   Bleeding; the escape of blood from arteries or veins in any part of the body. A haemorrhage can appear as a bruise.

Heparin   A naturally occurring substance found in many body tissues which inhibits the clotting of blood. Heparin injected into the body will help to prevent thrombosis.

Hirsutism   Excessive hairiness. The development of hair in women in places where it is normally only found in men.

Hormone   A chemical substance produced in one part of the body which passes via the bloodstream to another part where it has its effect. Different hormones control different functions within the body.

Hormone replacement therapy (HRT)   Treatment with drugs which attempts to replace, or partially replace, the hormones whose levels decline around the time of the menopause.

Hypothalamus   Part of the brain which, amongst other functions, is involved in hormone production.

Hysterectomy   The surgical removal of the uterus.

Hysteroscopy The insertion of a small telescope into the uterus which allows the surgeon to see inside it. The process is used to inspect the uterine cavity and to detect fibroids, polyps or cancer within it.

Incision A cut or wound made by a sharp instrument, such as during an operation.

Incontinence Lack of control of the discharge of urine or faeces.

Induction agent A drug which induces sleep.

Inhalational anaesthetic A drug in the form of a gas which is breathed in through a face mask.

Intermenstrual bleeding Bleeding between periods at times when it would not normally occur in the menstrual cycle.

Intoxication syndrome A condition involving mental confusion and possibly heart failure which can result from the body's absorption of too much water and sodium during surgery. It is a risk during operations such as endometrial resection when fluid is introduced into the uterine cavity to distend it.

Intra-uterine contraceptive device See **Coil**.

Intravenous anaesthetic An anaesthetic which is introduced into the body by injection into a vein.

Introitus The opening to the vagina in the vulva.

Labia (singular **labium**) The lip-shaped folds of skin around the external openings of the vagina and urethra.

Laparoscope A telescope-like instrument with a light source and camera attached which can be introduced into the abdominal cavity. It allows the surgeon to examine the internal organs without the need for a large incision to be made.

Laparoscopic sterilisation Sterilisation carried out with the aid of a laparoscope.

Laparoscopically assisted hysterectomy The surgical removal of the uterus which is done with the aid of a laparoscope.

Laparotomy An operation in which a long incision is made in the abdomen so that the surgeon can see into the abdominal cavity.

Ligament   A band of fibrous tissue connecting bones; or a strand of peritoneum which connects the abdominal organs to each other or to the abdominal wall. The **broad ligament** is attached to either side of the uterus and to the ovaries.

Linear stapler   An instrument which automatically staples and cuts tissue. The metal staples secure the cut ends of the tissue to prevent excessive blood loss.

Lithotomy position   A position used for some gynaecological operations in which the woman is placed on her back with her legs apart and her feet resting in stirrups.

Local anaesthetic   A drug which blocks the sensation in the area around which it is injected, causing numbness.

Luteinising hormone (LH)   The hormone produced by the pituitary gland in the brain and involved in the process of ovulation.

Luteinising hormone-releasing hormone (LHRH)   The hormone which stimulates the release of luteinising hormone.

Maintenance agent   A drug which keeps you asleep.

Medical history   Details of someone's past health, including illnesses, operations, allergies etc.

Menarche   The beginning of menstruation which occurs in girls at puberty, usually between the ages of 10 and 16 in the UK.

Menopause   The time at which spontaneous menstruation ceases in women at the end of their natural reproductive life.

Menorrhagia   Heavy or prolonged menstrual bleeding.

Menstrual cycle   The approximately monthly pattern of bleeding and the days between episodes of bleeding. Day 1 of the menstrual cycle is the day on which bleeding starts, and the last day is the day before the start of the next episode of bleeding. If heavy bleeding is preceded by very light bleeding or spotting, it is the first day of the heavy bleeding which is day 1 of the cycle.

Menstruation   The discharge of blood from the uterus which occurs at approximately monthly intervals in women throughout their reproductive life but which ceases during pregnancy and lactation.

Metrorrhagia   Irregular uterine bleeding.

Monitoring device   A piece of equipment which is used to watch over the various activities of the body, such as the heart beat, breathing rate etc.

Myomectomy   The surgical removal of fibroids from the uterus.

Myometrium   The muscle layer in the wall of the uterus.

Named nurse   A nurse allocated to a particular patient who is responsible for that patient's nursing care throughout their stay in hospital. The idea of 'named nurses' was introduced under the terms of the government's Patients' Charter.

'Nil by mouth'   A term used to mean that nothing – neither food nor drink – must be swallowed in the hours before an operation.

Non-absorbable suture/stitch   A stitch made of a material which will not dissolve. Non-absorbable sutures need to be removed once the wound has healed or, if they are used internally, remain in place forever.

Non-steroidal anti-inflammatory drug (NSAID)   A pain-killing drug which also helps reduce inflammation.

Norplant   A newly available contraceptive in the form of an implant, about the same size as a matchstick It can be inserted under the skin, usually in the arm, and releases progestogen into the body. It is effective for about 5 years and, when removed, fertility returns within a few days.

Obesity   An excessive amount of fat in the body. (Obesity is a non-specific term which is being replaced by a figure calculated from height and weight measurements and known as the **body mass index** (BMI).)

Obstetric history   Details of a woman's childbearing history, including how many children she has had, what the births were like, etc.

Obstetrician   A doctor who specialises in the care of women during pregnancy, childbirth and the period immediately after childbirth.

Oedema   Swelling of part of the body due to the accumulation in the tissues of fluid which has leaked from tiny blood vessels.

Oestrogen   A hormone which in women stimulates sexual development at puberty and changes in the endometrium during the menstrual cycle. It is produced by the ovaries and by the adrenal glands situated above the kidneys.

Oophorectomy   The surgical removal of an ovary.

Oral contraception   A method of contraception which involves taking pills by mouth.

Osteoporosis   A condition common in older women in which the bones become brittle and porous due to loss of minerals from them.

Ovarian cyst   A fluid-filled swelling which enlarges the ovary. Small ovarian cysts – up to 3 to 4 cm (1 to 1.5 inches) in diameter – are normal, and common. Larger ones can cause problems and may have to be surgically removed by **cystectomy**.

Ovarian follicle   A small cavity containing an ovum which is produced in an ovary.

Ovary   A female reproductive organ which produces ova and hormones.

Ovulation   The release of an ovum. Ovulation occurs 14 days before the start of the next period.

Ovulatory bleeding   Bleeding associated with ovulation.

Ovum   (plural: **ova**) A female egg before it has been fertilised by a sperm.

Palpitation   Increase in the heart rate due to exercise, anxiety or disease.

Paralytic ileus   Paralysis of the bowel which can occur following surgery.

Pelvis/Pelvic cavity   The cavity between the lower abdomen and groin which contains the bladder, lower rectum and some reproductive organs. (The pelvis is also the name given to the basin-shaped ring of bone which forms the hips.)

Period   The days of the menstrual cycle on which bleeding occurs.

Peritoneum   The membrane which lines the abdominal cavity and the upper pelvic cavity. It also forms a layer over the organs within these cavities.

Physiotherapist   Someone trained to help people to use physical exercise to correct deformities, restore function of a part of the body following injury or disease, and to build up the body's physical strength.

Pituitary gland   A gland at the base of the brain which secretes various hormones.

Polyp   A swelling on a stalk arising from the surface of the body or from an organ, such as the uterus.

Post-menopausal bleeding   Bleeding which occurs after the menopause, when menstrual bleeding should have ceased. Bleeding is classified as post-menopausal when it occurs at least 1 year after the last period.

Post-operative   After an operation.

Pouch of Douglas   A pocket between the vagina and rectum.

Premature menopause   Menopause which occurs spontaneously, i.e. not due to drug or surgical treatment, before the age of 40.

Premedication (premed.)   Any drug which is given before another, e.g. a drug given before an anaesthetic to reduce the patient's anxiety by making them more relaxed and drowsy.

Premenstrual tension (PMT)   An exacerbation of the normal changes in emotional and physical feelings which can occur prior to a menstrual period. Women often experience bloating, and swollen and sometimes tender breasts. They may cry or become angry more easily than usual.

Pre-operative   Before an operation.

Primary bleeding   Bleeding that occurs during an operation.

Procidentia   Prolapse of the uterus in which it protrudes through the external opening of the vagina.

Progesterone A steroid which stimulates changes in the female reproductive organs, preparing them for pregnancy. The main changes are an increase in the blood supply in the lining of the womb so that it can support a fetus. There may also be a slight increase in the size of the breasts.

Progestogen Any drug which mimics the action of progesterone.

Prolapse Sinking down of a part; prolapse of the uterus involves the sinking of the cervix into the vagina. More severe prolapse (**procidentia**) can result in the whole of the uterus protruding through the external opening of the vagina. Prolapse of the vagina is often associated with uterine prolapse, and involves descent of the walls of the vagina.

Puberty The time at which the sex glands become active. In girls, menstruation begins, the uterus, ovaries and vagina enlarge, and the breasts and pubic hair start to develop.

Pulmonary embolism A clot of blood or air bubble which forms within the blood vessels of the lungs.

Purgative A substance which aids the emptying of the bowels.

Pus A liquid produced as a result of inflammation. It contains both dead and living tissue fragments, cells and bacteria.

Pyrexia A fever.

Recovery room A ward near the operating theatre where patients are taken to recover from the anaesthetic after surgery. The recovery room is staffed by nurses who are specially trained in this type of care.

Rectum The last part of the large intestine between the colon and anus.

Resection The cutting out of part of an organ or tissue.

Resectoscope A telescope which bears an attachment for cutting tissue.

Retroverted uterus This is a normal, but less commonly found orientation of the uterus, the tip of which bends backwards towards the rectum and bowel.

Salpingo-oophorectomy The surgical removal of a fallopian tube (also known as a **salpinx**) together with an ovary.

Secondary bleeding Bleeding which occurs after an operation.

Secondary infection Infection occurring in an open wound while it is healing.

Sedative A drug which slows down the activity of a part or the whole of the body.

Side-effect An unwanted effect that accompanies another disease or treatment.

Sign Something a doctor looks for as evidence of disease or medical abnormality, for example swelling or bleeding.

Speculum Any instrument used to inspect a passage or tube, commonly the vagina.

Spinal anaesthetic A drug which is injected between the bones of the spine into the space around the nerves, and which causes numbness in the legs and lower abdomen.

Step-down ward A ward to which day-case patients go in some hospitals to recover before going home after an operation.

Sterilisation Sterilisation of women involves placing a clip or ring on the fallopian tubes to disrupt the passage of ova and sperm, and thus prevent conception from taking place.

Sterilisation is also a process of killing germs, particularly bacteria.

Subcutaneous Under the surface of the skin.

Sub-total hysterectomy The surgical removal of the body of the uterus, leaving the cervix in place.

Suppository A cone-shaped medical preparation, made of wax or gelatine and containing a drug, which can be inserted into the body, usually the rectum. Although solid at room temperature, the suppository melts at the temperature of the body.

Surgery The treatment of disease or injury by operation.

Suture A surgical stitch or row of stitches.

Symptom A disturbance to the normal working of the body which is not necessarily visible but is felt by the patient, for example pain or tiredness.

Threshold bleeding A very small amount of bleeding resulting from low levels of oestrogen and an absence of progesterone.

Thrombo-embolic deterrent stockings (TEDS) See **Anti-embolism stockings**

Thrombosis The coagulation of blood within a vein or artery to produce a blood clot.

Thrombus A blood clot which forms in, and remains in, a blood vessel or the heart.

Transcervical resection of the endometrium The surgical removal of the endometrial lining of the uterus by an instrument inserted through the cervix.

Transfusion See **Blood transfusion**

Trocar A sharp instrument which acts as a piloting instrument through which others can be inserted into a body cavity.

Tumour A swelling.

Umbilicus The navel.

Urethra The tube through which urine passes as it is discharged from the bladder. In women, the urethra is short, about 4 cm long, whereas in men it is much longer (18 to 20 cm).

Urinary retention The inability to empty the bladder.

Uterine perforation Damage which results in a hole being made in the wall of the uterus and which can occur accidentally during surgery.

Uterus The muscular organ in which an embryo develops during pregnancy; the womb.

Vagina The canal between the uterus and the vulva.

Vaginal hysterectomy The surgical removal of the uterus via the vagina.

Vulva The external female organs, including the openings of the vagina and urethra, the clitoris and the labia.

Warfarin An anticoagulant which can be administered to help prevent the blood coagulating and forming clots.

Womb The uterus.

How to complain

If you are unhappy about anything that has occurred – or, indeed, that has not occurred – during your stay in hospital, there are several possible paths to follow if you want to make a complaint.

However, before you set the complaints machinery in motion, you should give careful thought to what is involved. Once a formal complaint has been made against a doctor and the complaints procedure has begun, there is little chance of stopping it.

If you think you have a genuine grievance, do try to talk to the person concerned, explaining as clearly and unemotionally as possible what it is that you feel has gone wrong. If you do not feel able to discuss things directly, you can always present your case in a letter.

The vast majority of doctors – GPs and hospital doctors – are dedicated, conscientious and hard working. They really do have their patients' best interests at heart, and many work very long hours each week, night and day. Junior hospital doctors, for example, may have to work 80 hours or more a week, their overtime being compulsory and poorly paid.

A complaint against a doctor is usually a devastating blow, which can cause considerable stress. Of course, if something has gone wrong during your medical treatment, you may also have suffered stress and unhappiness, but before you make an official complaint, do consider whether your doctor's actions have really warranted what many would see as a 'kick in the teeth'.

The best approach is to make a polite and reasoned enquiry to the person concerned. However angry or irritated you may feel, you are likely to find that a complaint made aggressively – however justified this may seem – is unlikely to achieve much.

Leaflets and other information giving details of all the appropriate councils and complaints procedures and how they work can be obtained from your hospital or local health authority. Your local Citizens' Advice Bureau or Community Health Council will also be able to give you information about what to do and who to go to for help if you have any problems with the offices mentioned here.

Hospital staff

If your complaint concerns something that has happened during your stay in hospital, and for some reason you are unable to approach the person directly concerned, you can talk to the ward sister or charge nurse, the hospital doctor on your ward, or the senior manager for the department or ward. Many complaints can be dealt with directly by one of these people, but if this is not possible, they will be able to refer you to the appropriate person.

The General Manager

If you are intimidated by the thought of speaking to one of the people mentioned above, you can write to the hospital's General Manager, sometimes called the Director of Operations or Chief Executive. The General Manager has responsibility for the way the hospital is run.

The Government's Patients' Charter states that anyone making a complaint about an NHS service must receive a 'full and prompt written reply from the Chief Executive or General Manager'. You should therefore receive an immediate response to your letter, and your complaint should be fully investigated by a senior manager.

The hospital switchboard, or any medical or clerical staff at the hospital, should be able to give you the General Manager's name and office address. If you would prefer to do so, you can make an appointment to speak to him or her, rather than writing a letter.

Depending on how serious your complaint is, you should receive either a full report of the investigation into it, or regular letters telling you what is happening until such a report can be made.

Do make sure you keep copies of all letters you write and receive concerning your complaint.

District Health Authority

If the treatment you require is not available in your area, or the waiting list is very long, you can contact your local District Health Authority. The District Health Authority is able to deal with complaints concerning the provision of services, rather than with those resulting from something going wrong with your treatment. The District Health Authority can sometimes arrange for you to have treatment elsewhere where waiting lists are shorter if this is what you want.

Your NHS authority should produce a leaflet to explain how it deals with complaints. This will be available at your hospital or clinic. If you have any difficulty finding out who to contact, write to the general manager of the hospital. The hospital will be able to tell you which health authority covers the area in which you live.

Community Health Council

If you feel that you would like independent advice and assistance, you can obtain this from your local Community Health

Council. Someone from the Community Health Council will be able to explain the complaints procedures to you, help you to write letters to the hospital, and also come with you to any meetings arranged between hospital representatives and yourself. Again, the address of the Community Health Council for your area can be obtained from a hospital or local telephone directory.

Regional Medical Officer

If your complaint concerns the standard of *clinical* treatment you received in hospital, and the paths you have already taken have not led to a satisfactory conclusion, you can take it to the Regional Medical Officer for your area.

Family Health Services Authority

Any complaint about a GP which you have been unable to sort out with the doctor in question can be reported to the Family Health Services Authority. Such complaints should be made within 13 weeks of the incident occurring. Again, your local Community Health Council will be able to give you advice, help you make your complaint, and help you to write letters etc.

Health Service Commissioner

If all else has failed, you can take your complaint to the Health Service Commissioner, who deals with complaints made by individuals against the NHS. The Commissioner is independent of both the NHS and the government, being responsible to Parliament.

The Health Service Commissioner is able to deal with complaints concerning the failure of a NHS authority to provide the service it should – a failure which has caused you actual hardship or injustice. However, you must have taken your complaint up with your local health authority first. If you have not received a satisfactory response within a reasonable time, you must enclose copies of *all* the relevant letters and documents as well as giving details of the incident itself when writing to the Health Service Commissioner. The Health Commissioner is not able to investigate complaints about clinical treatment.

You must also contact the Health Service Commissioner within *one* year of the incident occurring, unless there is some valid reason why you have been unable to do so.

There is a separate Health Service Commissioner for each country within the United Kingdom.

Health Service Commissioner for England
Church House
Great Smith Street
London SW1P 3BW
Telephone: 071 276 2035

Health Service Commissioner for Scotland
Second Floor
11 Melville Crescent
Edinburgh EH3 7LU
Telephone: 031 225 7465

Health Service Commissioner for Wales
4th Floor Pearl Assurance House
Greyfriars Road
Cardiff CF1 3AG
Telephone: 0222 394621

Office of the Northern Ireland Commissioner for Complaints
33 Wellington Place
Belfast BT1 6HN
Telephone: 0232 233821

Taking legal action

The legal path is likely to be an expensive one, and should be a last resort rather than a starting point.

In theory, everyone has a right to take legal action. However, unless you have very little money and are entitled to Legal Aid, or a great deal of money, you are unlikely to be able to afford this costly process. The outcome of legal action can never be assured, and the possible cost if you lose your case should be borne in mind.

If you do think you have grounds for compensation for injury caused to you as a result of negligence, advice can be sought from:

The Association for the Victims of Medical Accidents (AVMA)
1 London Road
Forest Hill
London SE23 3TP
Telephone: 081 291 2793.

Someone from the AVMA will be able to give you free and confidential legal advice about whether or not you have a case worth pursuing. They will also be able to recommend solicitors with training in medical law who may be prepared to represent you.

Summary

Do tell nursing or other medical staff if you are not happy about *any* aspect of your care in hospital. They may be able to deal with your complaint immediately. But do remember, if your complaint is about a serious matter, or if you are not satisfied with the response you receive, you are entitled to pursue it through all the levels that exist to deal with such problems.

Index